T0259698

SpringerBriefs in Well-Being and Quality of Life Research

SpringerBriefs in Well-Being and Quality-of-Life Research are concise summaries of cutting-edge research and practical applications across the field of well-being and quality of life research. These compact refereed monographs are under the editorial supervision of an international Advisory Board*. Volumes are 50 to 125 pages (approximately 20,000–70,000 words), with a clear focus. The series covers a range of content from professional to academic such as: snapshots of hot and/or emerging topics, in-depth case studies, and timely reports of state-of-the art analytical techniques. The scope of the series spans the entire field of Well-Being Research and Quality-of-Life Studies, with a view to significantly advance research. The character of the series is international and interdisciplinary and will include research areas such as: health, cross-cultural studies, gender, children, education, work and organizational issues, relationships, job satisfaction, religion, spirituality, ageing from the perspectives of sociology, psychology, philosophy, public health and economics in relation to Well-being and Quality-of-Life research. Volumes in the series may analyze past, present and/or future trends, as well as their determinants and consequences. Both solicited and unsolicited manuscripts are considered for publication in this series. SpringerBriefs in Well-Being and Quality-of-Life Research will be of interest to a wide range of individuals with interest in quality of life studies, including sociologists, psychologists, economists, philosophers, health researchers, as well as practitioners across the social sciences. Briefs will be published as part of Springer's eBook collection, with millions of users worldwide. In addition, Briefs will be available for individual print and electronic purchase. Briefs are characterized by fast, global electronic dissemination, standard publishing contracts, easy-to-use manuscript preparation and formatting guidelines, and expedited production schedules. We aim for publication 8–12 weeks after acceptance. Both solicited and unsolicited manuscripts are considered for publication in this series.

More information about this series at http://www.springer.com/series/10150

Janet L. Currie

Managing Motherhood

A New Wellness Perspective

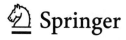 Springer

Janet L. Currie
Faculty of Arts and Social Sciences, School
   of Education and International Studies
University of Technology Sydney
Sydney, NSW
Australia

ISSN 2211-7644   ISSN 2211-7652   (electronic)
SpringerBriefs in Well-Being and Quality of Life Research
ISBN 978-981-13-0337-1   ISBN 978-981-13-0338-8   (eBook)
https://doi.org/10.1007/978-981-13-0338-8

Library of Congress Control Number: 2018939309

Printed on acid-free paper

This Springer imprint is published by the registered company Springer Nature Singapore Pte Ltd.
part of Springer Nature
The registered company address is: 152 Beach Road, #21-01/04 Gateway East, Singapore 189721,
Singapore

Foreword

I'm lucky enough to have known Dr. Janet L. Currie from our days as young athletes when our mums would drive us to sport practices after school, have all the right foods, clothes washed and ready for us, and be our everything as teens growing up in the 1970s. Janet has continued on a path of research and personal discovery while continuing to share her learning on how to keep a positive attitude through her own journey of work, life, and motherhood.

With Janet as a constant inspiration in my life, I was then honored to lecture teaching methods at UTS under her guidance as head lecturer and again learned more lifelong lessons from her on how I can balance my own life and find thankfulness for what I have and in turn happiness at every turn.

In life, coping means having the resilience to utilize our strengths and master situations. In doing so, it builds our sense of confidence, self-worth, and self-esteem. When we become new mothers ourselves, we're not always sure what to do; however, with the anticipated guidance possible from reading *Managing Motherhood*, women and practitioners can now gain ready access to healthy ideas on positive strategies and tips of how to cope with this challenging role. In the book, Janet talks about how the mothers say there can be different levels or degrees of coping. However, Janet provides evidence to show it is more than simply 'putting up' with a bad situation. Instead, Janet writes, it is demonstrating daily how we can conquer challenges and live in a positive way, therefore building individual mental health. Janet's book helps each individual develop a sense of subjective well-being giving strength to those women knowing how to rise above the pressures of perfect images and behaviors and know that it is more than all right to ask for support.

To access the data for *Managing Motherhood*, Janet spoke in depth with mothers of young children to gain their insights and ideas. Her research is therefore grounded in reality and has meaning based on real-life experiences. With the support and guidance I have learned from Janet along with the knowledge I have gained from others, education, Neuro Linguistic Programming and the Olympic Journey, I feel honored to now live a life in Hawaii and around the world of happiness and love. I get to wake up every morning with a passion for life, a thankfulness for what I have and an excitement for assisting others to find the same in their 'own' journey and day-to-day life situations.

Janet is a dedicated, thorough researcher and has looked at this topic from many angles to provide great insight, knowledge, and confidence to support every woman navigating the journey of motherhood, relationships, and life, with no 'how to guidebooks' coming with your own situations or children.

This book gives a wonderful strength to everyone who reads it through giving us skills in finding the perspective that can always find the good in all people, relationships, and any situation that presents itself.

Honolulu, USA   Shelley Oates–Wilding

Contents

Keywords Mothers · Coping · Coping strategies · Wellness · Wellbeing Health · Resilience · Subjective wellness · Women · Lifestyle Mental health

Chapter 1
Introduction

Abstract The first few years of motherhood can be a stressful and challenging time for mothers. Mothers need to manage this period positively to reduce the amount of stress and feel in control. Coping strategies used by mothers of young children is an important area to explore because feeling in control of one's environment has important consequences for health, well-being, and feelings of confidence and adequacy in the motherhood role. Past research has also demonstrated that anxious mothers are less satisfied with quality of life and their motherhood role. From a wellness perspective, effective coping depends on an individual's personal evaluation of the situation. However, there is limited research available explaining what this means from the mother's own perspective. Much of the existing research on women's mental health has not clarified the nature of the coping experience from a subjective wellness perspective, nor taken a grounded theory approach using the participant's own words and meanings to describe the experience. Consequently, there are limited insights as to how it should be understood, defined and achieved. Well or healthy mothers constitute the majority of the population, however, the focus of past research has been on 'not-coping', marginalised groups, or unhealthy approaches. *Managing Motherhood* was written to provide enlightenment on the nature and meaning of the coping experience for new mothers, and insight to the strategies they use to maintain feelings of subjective wellbeing. This chapter contains definitions of key terms, limitations in interpreting the findings, and outlines the book's chapters.

1.1 Background to *Managing Motherhood*

The period of early motherhood can represent a period of great stress, change and personal demands within a woman's life (Bishop, 1999; McVeigh, 1998; Rowe, Temple, & Hawthorne, 1996). Common problems experienced by new mothers may include concerns for the baby's health, anxiety, lifestyle changes, depression, relationship problems, lack of support or personal health. Social and financial factors often compound the problems faced by new mothers (Rowe et al., 1996).

© The Author(s) 2018
J. L. Currie, *Managing Motherhood*, SpringerBriefs in Well-Being and Quality
of Life Research, https://doi.org/10.1007/978-981-13-0338-8_1

Social factors include low self-esteem, previous physical or emotional abuse, social isolation, lack of emotional support from partners or lack of access to information on how to "draw on positive ways of coping" (Rowe et al., 1996, p. S56). Financial difficulties can affect coping because mothers may be deterred from seeking out health and medical services or other resources and assistance.

Mothers may also feel stressed because they may identify themselves as having primary responsibility for childcare. The ideology of motherhood suggests that mothers should be selfless, nurturing, coping and available at all times (Wearing, 1984). Harris (1998) noted that this sense of sole responsibility by the mother and the dependence of the family on her can mean she is more reluctant to seek out help or engage the strategy of social support in order to cope. However, Wearing (1984) and Harris (1998) both pointed out that middle class mothers may relate more to feminist ideals and be therefore more likely to balance their own needs amongst those of other family members. Wearing (1984) described this phenomenon as being less "completely defined" by the demands of motherhood.

A central issue of concern is how mothers cope with their new role and what strategies they implement in order to feel in control. Much of the past research has focused on definitions and classifications of types of coping. Coping is the effort required to deal with difficult experiences (Musil & Abraham, 1986) while Scherk (1999, p. 24) believes that, "coping involves the many things people think, say, and do to reduce, mitigate, master, or tolerate the demands of stressful circumstances". Coping behaviours are often classified as emotional or problem-focused coping (Lazarus & Folkman, 1984; Scherk, 1999), with problem-focused, active coping styles or strategies shown to be more effective in dealing with stress than avoidance or withdrawal mechanisms (Goldsmith-Cwikel, Dielman, Kirscht, & Israel, 1988). However, Harris (1998, p. 2) found it more useful to identify mothers' coping strategies in terms of "norms of reciprocity and social distance". That is, a mother is most likely to select strategies that incur the least reciprocal obligation, such as coping by herself, or paying for a cleaner.

Coping strategies used by mothers of young children is an important area to investigate because feeling in control of one's environment has important consequences for health, well-being, and feelings of confidence and adequacy in the motherhood role (Fowles, 1998). Coping strategies or personal efforts subjectively evaluated as being effective, usually result in an individual feeling a greater sense of control. This is due to the positive sense of social competence and self-esteem they feel which positively affects health (Goldsmith-Cwikel et al., 1988, p. 170).

1.2 Significance of the Research

It has been widely reported in the literature that motherhood can be a very stressful experience and transitional period (Fairbrother, Janssen, Antony, Tucker, & Young, 2016; Maushart, 1997; Raphael-Leff, 1993; Sethi, 1995), with the first three years of motherhood considered the most labour-exhaustive (Walker & Wilging, 2000).

Coping consists of efforts to manage such stressors or control difficult experiences (Monat & Lazarus, 1985). Investigating coping strategies is justified as it helps eluci-date how mothers deal with stressors. Effective coping strategies can help to reduce stress levels (Currie, 2009; Scherk, 1999) and "control one's experiences" (Musil & Abraham, 1986, p. 194). Mothers need to be able to draw upon suitable strategies to reduce the risk of experiencing anxiety and depression (Rowe et al., 1996).

Little is known about the process of coping and what the strategies entail (Musil & Abraham, 1986). Strategies vary between individuals with similar or dissimilar problems (Pearlin, 1985). Effective coping depends on the individual's evaluation of the situation. Much of the existing research on women's mental health has not clarified the nature of the coping experience, nor taken a grounded theory approach using the participant's own words and meanings to describe the experience. Research has tended to focus on coping within marginalised groups using ill or disadvantaged samples (Aftyka, Rybojad, Rosa, Wróbel, & Karakuła-Juchnowicz, 2017; Kolotylo & Broome, 2000; Kvarme, Alebertini Früh, & Lidèn, 2017; Nelson, Miles, & Belyea, 1997; Sharts-Hopko, Regan-Kubinsko, Lincoln, & Heverly, 1996; Tein, Sandler, & Zantra, 2000). Well or healthy mothers constitute the majority of the population, however, the focus has been on 'not-coping', or ineffective coping and unhealthy approaches. More research is needed on identifying the strategies mothers use to maintain their own perception of coping (Luthar, 2015; Razurel, Kaiser, Sellenet, & Epiney, 2013). In addition, according to Pridham (1997), theoretical constructions concerning the nature of strategies important in the context of day-to-day coping are needed to describe and explain how the coping phenomenon might occur.

This book bridges a gap in the literature by examining mothers' own descriptions of their coping symptoms and strategies, in the context of their everyday lives. As in-depth research into the lived experiences of mothers can provide rich descriptions about their experiences and the ideological contexts of their mothering that more wide ranging research can only hint at (Harris, 1998, p. 5). Scepticism has also been raised about the value of forced-choice measures or inventories for the objective or subjective examination of coping (Kobus & Reyes, 2000; McVeigh, 1998). These quantitative tools cannot record a person's own thoughts or perspectives about every-day coping or coping strategies (Goldsmith-Cwikel et al., 1988; Taylor & Aspinwall, 1996). The 'reality' of inventories, externally administered by a researcher, may in fact be meaningless to the rich descriptions able to be supplied by the individual research participant (Im, 2000). Coping does not have to be 'objectively' measured. Effective coping outcomes only require a belief or subjective feeling by the indi-vidual that one is in control. Further, the situational examples used in standardised coping measurement tools may not be applicable to a mother's lifestyle or setting (Hart, 1996). In-depth interviewing may provide a more complete understanding of the coping process.

The coping strategies nominated by the mothers in this book may be recommended in terms of anticipatory guidance, for example, to assist others to cope with stress. The research helps guide professional practice by offering strategies other mothers may find useful in similar situations. Comprehensive health care should consider each woman's unique experience (Sethi, 1995).

1.3 Definition of Terms

The following definitions used throughout the book arise from commonly accepted and standard health promotion terminology and discourse:

Coping: feeling in control of one's situation, a perception of handling stressors effectively or adequately. A personal perception of 'managing motherhood'.

Coping strategies: the methods or particular efforts utilised by a mother in order to cope or deal with day-to-day life experiences. What mothers do to 'manage motherhood'.

Hardiness: a robust feeling of having adequate personal coping skills available to deal with day-to-day stressors. Confidently viewing stressful daily situations as challenges to be overcome.

Health: Experiencing a balanced state of individual physical, mental, social and spritual well-being. Related to feelings of coping and a sense of control of one's environment.

Lifestyle: the combination of behaviours or way of life that a mother acquires, affected by social, physical, mental, cultural and environmental influences.

Managing Motherhood: a new wellness perspective of mothers' coping; developing a set of coping strategies to resiliently face and overcome daily challenges and events, and maintain a sense of subjective wellness.

Motherhood: the experiences encountered by a mother in her role or day-to-day lifestyle.

Mental health: a sense of social and emotional well-being; a feeling of coping and being able to realistically manage and enjoy daily living.

Resilience: the ability to 'bounce back' from or cope with major life changes or stressors. Holding or building the strengths, resources and capabilities to adapt, adjust, recover and grow following the personal experience of individual setbacks, adverse events and challenges.

Stress: an individual's physical and mental reaction to stressors, including anxiety, tension, worry or events.

Stressor: any external situations or events placing demands on an individual.

Subjective Wellness: an individual's own perceived sense of experiencing a positive state of well-being.

Well-being: achieving a balanced state of the mental, physical, social and spiritual aspects of individual health; feeling a sense of mental health and coping with the normal stresses of life.

1.4 Aims and Purpose of the Book

The purpose of writing *Managing Motherhood* was to report on the outcomes of my in-depth qualitative study researching the strategies mothers of young children use to cope with their everyday lifestyle. The book explains the methods or strengths mothers use when coping with day-to-day experiences. This research values the individual perspectives a group of informants provided on their mothering experiences. In this way, any theory has been built upon information supplied by the women of their own unique experiences.

1.5 Research Question

The research question that was used to focus the direction and scope of the book is, "What strategies do well mothers of young children 0–5 years utilise in order to feel that they are coping with their everyday lifestyle?" In addressing this research question during the natural course of the investigation, three sub-questions became apparent:

1. What is the meaning of the coping experience?
2. What situations do mothers feel they need to cope with?
3. What strategies do mothers use to deal with these situations?

1.6 Limitations

Coping is a complex process influenced by a variety of factors (Naughton, 1997). It is the effort required to adapt to some sort of stressor or external demand. Motherhood is generally viewed as a stressful period (Littlewood & McHugh, 1997), however individual perceptions of the degree of this stress, including one's ability to cope, are influenced by a range of factors:

1. Personal judgement (Bolger, 1990)
2. Resources and environment (Mattlin, Wethington, & Kessler, 1990)
3. Culture (Lazarus, 1996).

Coping involves a primary appraisal of whether a stressor is viewed as a threat, loss, challenge or not very stressful at all. That is, stressors are judged 'through the eye of the beholder' when the individual asks, "How stressful is this situation?". It is important to note that what is viewed as threatening to one person may appear neutral or non-challenging to another. This book has explored situations mothers felt they have to cope with, but did not attempt to rate or quantify comparative levels of stress between respondents.

The success of one's coping efforts is most effectively judged by the individual (McCrae, Costa, & Zonderman, 1994). However, an individual could hold too high an expectation, be unrealistic, or repressively deny that they are not coping (Duff, 1997). The research undertaken for this book did not investigate whether respondents were deluded in feeling that they had 'effectively' coped with stress. It did not use inventories and seek that the mothers complete those to objectively evaluate coping outcomes. Nor were external 'experts' employed to assess a mother's coping situation. Rather, this book is underpinned by the health promoting view that the key feature is whether the mothers themselves feel that they are coping and in control of their situation. This forms a new wellness perspective of coping. It is one which places the control and the most empowered position with a mother herself. She is in control of her environment, perceptions and expressions.

Nevertheless, it has to be acknowledged that personal judgements of coping outcomes can be affected by personality. McCrae, Costa, and Zonderman (1994, p. 2) concluded that "coping is personality in action under stress". Individuals high in neuroticism may react badly to stress, blame themselves or become withdrawn. Extraverts may be able to relate to others and talk more under stress (Taylor & Aspinwall, 1996). Hardiness can be defined as how well an individual 'handles' stress. It includes having a sense of control and commitment, and viewing stress as a challenge (Naughton, 1997). Type A personalities tend to be more competitive, impatient and hostile than Type Bs who are more relaxed and uncompetitive. Type Cs tend to repress or ignore stress (Cinelli & Ziegler, 1990). Individuals with attachment styles who tend to want to please others constantly may be more likely to adopt the 'supermum' approach and try to cope with 'everything', rather than negotiate or say "no" (Alexander, Feeney, Noller, & Hohaus, 1998; Raskin, Kummel, & Bannister, 1998).

This book contains in-depth descriptions by mothers of the strategies they implement in their efforts to cope with or handle stressors. However, psychological measurements of the effects of personality on coping ability, such as degrees of level of 'Type A' or 'B', optimism, pessimism, hardiness, relationship and attachment styles, were not employed.

Individual perceptions of the influence of one's environment or accessibility of available resources can affect coping or degree of self-efficacy. This is the belief or confidence in one's own ability to fulfil a task (Alexander et al., 1998; Mattlin, Wethington, & Kessler, 1990). According to Lazarus and Folkman (1984), coping involves a secondary appraisal or evaluation of what coping resources are available in order to deal with what has been considered (primarily) as a stressful situation. Resources include health levels and energy, problem-solving skills, social skills and support, and material or financial resources. The study did not attempt to objectively measure levels of resources available such as problem-solving ability, social support, or levels of resourcefulness and help-seeking behaviour. Further, the study did not attempt to investigate any effect that socio-economic differences may have had on the coping strategies used. It is an assumption of this study that all respondents perceive that they are well. Respondents were not experiencing a chronic illness, and were living in reasonably stable conditions with access to social support (Alexander et al., 1998).

Coping is affected by cultural expectations and gender roles (Frankenhauser, 1994). Women are socialised to be feminine, silent and persevere under pressure. Some older studies showed that individuals with more androgynous than feminine mothering styles may tend to employ problem-solving techniques (Levo, 1983; Reilly, 1981).

Some individual mothers may wish to perceive themselves as coping effectively and well adjusted, especially in front of others. It has been widely reported in the literature that there is wide social pressure on mothers to be in control or at least keep up a 'façade' of 'I'm coping', because that's what 'good' mothers do (Dix, 1987). For the mothers in this study, this concept may be linked to the 'ideology of motherhood'—a 'good' mother is always available, unselfish, loving, understanding, calm and patient. Even when exhausted or without support, a mother must at all times be in complete control of her emotions; "The cardinal sin of motherhood with its associated guilt is to lose one's temper with a child…" (Wearing, 1984, p. 49). In this book I have attempted to explore respondents' identification with the ideological norm in terms of coping strategies. Even though all of the participating mothers live in a similar locality and share some common background, it was an assumption that they were exposed to similar ideological pressures.

The informants were limited to a purposeful sample of women who volunteered to take part in in-depth interviews. The sample is not quantitatively representative, limiting extrapolation of the results beyond this group of mothers. Nonetheless, the theoretical sampling technique used, and rich descriptions of situations, events, people and techniques, suggest that the coping experiences these mothers experienced may also apply to mothers in similar circumstances elsewhere.

1.7 Outline of the Book

Section I of *Managing Motherhood* contains the prologue. Chapter 2 details a profile of the research undertaken, including an account of the research design and method. Chapter 3 outlines the extent of current understanding in research on coping strategies used by mothers.

Section II of the book presents the main qualitative findings (Chaps. 4 and 5), and is devoted to discussing those results (Chap. 6). Chapter 7 unpacks factors identified by the mothers as having a major influence on their coping experience. Section III states the conclusions and recommendations, located in Chap. 8.

Chapter 2 outlines the research undertaken for *Managing Motherhood*, including an introduction to the mothers who participated.

References

Alexander, R., Feeney, J., Noller, P., & Hohaus, L. (1998). *Attachment style and coping resources as predictors of coping strategies in the transition to parenthood*. Melbourne: Australian Institute of Family Studies.

Aftyka, A., Rybojad, B , Rosa, W., Wróbel, A., & Karakuła-Juchnowicz, H. (2017). Risk factors for the development of post-traumatic stress disorder and coping strategies in mothers and fathers following infant hospitalisation in the neonatal intensive care unit. *Journal of Clinical Nursing, 26*, 4436–4445.

Bishop, L. (1999). *Postnatal depression: Families in turmoil.* Rushcutters Bay, Sydney: Halstead.

Bolger, N. (1990). Coping as a personality process: A prospective study. *Journal of Personality and Social Psychology, 59,* 525–537.

Cinelli, L. A., & Ziegler, D. J. (1990). Cognitive appraisal of daily hassles in college students showing Type A or Type B behavior patterns. *Psychological Reports, 67,* 83–88.

Currie, J. L. (2009). Managing motherhood: Strategies used by new mothers to maintain perceptions of wellness. *Health Care for Women International, 30,* 655–670.

Dix, C. (1987). *The new mother syndrome. Coping with postnatal stress and depression.* North Sydney: Allen and Unwin.

Duff, J. (1997). *Repressive denial, locus of control, and coping styles, and their relationships with immunosuppression, cardiovascular function and health outcomes.* Retrieved from http://www. adhd.com.au/immunity.html.

Fairbrother, N., Janssen, P., Antony, M. M., Tucker, E., & Young, A. H. (2016). Perinatal anxiety disorder prevalence and incidence. *Journal of Affective Disorders, 200,* 148–155.

Fowles, E. R. (1998). The relationship between maternal role attainment and postpartum depression. *Health Care for Women International, 19,* 83–94.

Frankenhauser, M. (1994). A biopsychosocial approach to stress in women and men. In V. J. Adesso, D. M. Reddy, & R. Fleming (Eds.), *Psychological perspectives on women's health* (pp. 39–56). Washington: Taylor & Francis.

Goldsmith-Cwikel, J. M., Dielman, T. E., Kirscht, J. P., & Israel, B. A. (1988). Mechanisms of psychosocial effects on health: The role of social integration, coping style and health behavior. *Health Education Quarterly, 15,* 151–173.

Harris, N. (1998). Coping with young children: how do mothers do it? In *Proceedings of the 6th Australian Institute of Family Studies (AIFS) Conference* (pp. 1–5). Melbourne: AIFS.

Hart, K. E. (1996). A comparison of two techniques for scoring episodic coping data. *Personality and Individual Differences, 21,* 159–162.

Im, E.-O. (2000). A feminist critique of research on women's work and health. *Health Care for Women International, 21,* 105–119.

Kobus, K., & Reyes, O. (2000). A descriptive study of urban mexican American adolescents' perceived stress and coping. *Hispanic Journal of Behavioral Science, 22,* 163–178.

Kolotylo, C. J., & Broome, M. E. (2000). Exploration of migraine pain, disability, depressive symptomatology, and coping: A pilot study. *Health Care for Women International, 21,* 203–218.

Kvarme, L. G., Alebertini Früh, E., & Lidèn, H. (2017). How do immigrant parents of children with complex health needs manage to cope in their daily lives? *Child and Family Social Work, 22,* 1399–1406.

Lazarus, R. S. (1996). The role of coping in the emotions and how coping changes over the life course. In C. Magai & S. H. McFadden (Eds.), *Handbook of emotions, adult development & aging* (pp. 289–306). San Diego: Academic.

Lazarus, R. S., & Folkman, S. (1984). *Stress, Appraisal and Coping.* New York: Springer.

Levo, L. M. (1983). An investigation of the efficacy of competing explanations of how women cope with stressful home-career conflicts. *Dissertation Abstracts International, 44-06B,* 1967.

Littlewood, J., & McHugh, N. (1997). *Maternal distress and postnatal depression. The myth of madonna.* Basingstoke, UK: Macmillan.

Luthar, S. S. (2015). Mothering Mothers. *Research in Human Development, 12,* 295–303.

Mattlin, J., Wethington, E., & Kessler, R. (1990). Situational determinants of coping and coping effectiveness. *Journal of Health and Social Behavior, 31,* 103–122.

Maushart, S. (1997). *The mask of motherhood. How motherhood changes everything and why we pretend it doesn't.* Milson's Point, Sydney: Random House.

McCrae, R. R, Costa, P. T., & Zonderman, A. B. (1994). *Stress, coping and personality in aging men and women* (online). Baltimore, USA: National Institute on Aging. Retrieved from http://axp1.grc.nia.nih.gov/1pc/1pcann/1994/180.html.

McVeigh, C. (1998). Functional status after childbirth in an Australian sample. *Journal of Obstetric, Gynecologic, and Neonatal Nursing, 27,* 402–409.

Monat, A., & Lazarus, R. S. (1985). Introduction: Stress and coping—Some current issues and controversies. In A. Monat, & R. S. Lazarus (Eds.), *Stress and coping. An anthology* (2nd ed., pp. 1–12). New York: Columbia.

Musil, C. M., & Abraham, I. L. (1986). Coping, thinking, and mental health nursing: Cognitions and their application to psychosocial intervention. *Issues in Mental Health Nursing, 8,* 191–210.

Naughton, F. O. (1997). *Stress and coping.* Northridge, USA: California State University. Retrieved from http://www.csun.edu/~vcpsy00h/students/coping.htm.

Nelson, A. E., Miles, M. S., & Belyea, M. J. (1997). Coping and support effects on mothers' stress responses to their child's hematopoietic stemcell transplantation. *Journal of Pediatric Oncology Nursing, 14,* 202–212.

Pearlin, L. I. (1985). Life strains and psychological distress among adults. In A. Monat, & R. S. Lazarus (Eds.), *Stress and coping. An anthology* (2nd ed., pp. 244–257). New York: Columbia.

Pridham, K. F. (1997). Mother's help-seeking as care initiated in a social context. *Image—The Journal of Nursing Scholarship, 29,* 65–70.

Raphael-Leff, J. (1993). *Psychological processes of childbearing.* London: Chapman & Hall.

Raskin, P. M., Kummel, P., & Bannister, T. (1998). The relationship between coping styles, attachment, and career salience in partnered working women with children. *Journal of Career Assessment, 6,* 403–416.

Razurel, C., Kaiser, B., Sellenet, C., & Epiney, M. (2013). Relation between perceived stress, social support, and coping strategies and maternal well-being: A review of the literature. *Women and Health, 53,* 74–99.

Reilly, S. J. (1981). The relation of sex-role orientation in women to coping style and cognitive response to stress. *Dissertation Abstracts International, 42-08B,* 3438.

Rowe, L., Temple, S., & Hawthorne, G. (1996). Mothers' emotional needs and difficulties after childbirth. *Clinical Psychologist, 25,* S53–S58.

Scherk, K. A. (1999). Recognizing coping behaviors. *American Journal of Nursing, 99,* 24–28.

Sethi, S. (1995). The dialectic in becoming a mother: Experiencing a postpartum phenomenon. *Scandinavian Journal of Caring Science, 9,* 235–244.

Sharts-Hopko, N. C., Regan-Kubinsko, M. J., Lincoln, P. S., & Heverly, M. A. (1996). Problem-focused coping in HIV-infected mothers in relation to self-efficacy, uncertainty, social support, and psychological distress. *IMAGE: Journal of Nursing Scholarship, 28,* 107–111.

Taylor, S. E., & Aspinwall, L. G. (1996). Mediating and moderating processes in psychosocial stress. In H. B. Kaplan (Ed.), *Psychosocial stress. Perspectives on structure, theory, life-course and methods* (pp. 71–110). San Diego, USA: Academic.

Tein, J.-Y., Sandler, I. N., & Zautra, A. J. (2000). Stressful life events, psychological distress, coping, and parenting of divorced mothers: A longitudinal study. *Journal of Family Psychology, 14,* 27–41.

Walker, L., & Wilging, S. (2000). Rediscovering the "M" in "MCH": Maternal health promotion after childbirth. *Journal of Obstetric, Gynaecologic and Neonatal Nursing, 29,* 229–236.

Wearing, B. (1984). *The ideology of motherhood.* Sydney: George Allen and Unwin.

Chapter 2
The Research Profile

Abstract Using a qualitative, grounded theory research approach, I utilised in-depth interviewing to discover the views and opinions of mothers about their lifestyles and coping experiences. This chapter contains a description of the informants, the theoretical underpinnings of the research, plus the techniques and methods used to access and analyse the data.

2.1 Description of the Research Methods Undertaken

This chapter describes how the main research informing the book was conducted and incorporates an explanation of the procedures involved.

2.1.1 Research Design

The research informing the data discussed in the book was originally conducted utilising a qualitative exploratory design with a grounded theory approach. "Grounded theory is a qualitative research approach used to explore the social processes that present within human interactions" (Carpenter, 1995, p. 145). A grounded theory research design is appropriate when investigating something for which little is known (Chenitz & Swanson, 1986; Minichiello, Fulton, & Sullivan, 1999; Punch, 1998). The unique grounded theory methodology used in *Managing Motherhood* is a highly systematic research approach often used for the purpose of understanding social and psychological phenomena.

The objective of grounded theory is the development of theory that explains basic patterns common in social life, such as the Coping Cycle, reported in Chap. 6. The grounded theory approach utilised in this book aligns with the view that any theory emerging from the study arises from the data itself, and not from some other source (Crotty, 1998). It is a process of inductive theory building, based squarely on the

© The Author(s) 2018
J. L. Currie, *Managing Motherhood*, SpringerBriefs in Well-Being and Quality of Life Research, https://doi.org/10.1007/978-981-13-0338-8_2

observation of the data themselves. With a grounded theory design, "one does not begin with a theory, then prove it" (Carpenter, 1995, p. 146). Instead, one starts with an area of study (such as coping strategies used by mothers of young children) and what is relevant to that area is allowed to emerge. Therefore, the findings can authentically inform professional practice in a patient-centred manner as the information and recommendations are in the words of 'real' mothers. This is in opposition to medical, 'top-down' approaches which attempt to explain well-being phenomena experienced by individuals.

2.1.2 The Participants

The main purpose of *Managing Motherhood* is to thoroughly detail coping strategies used by mothers of young children (0–5 years) to attain a sense of subjective wellness. As the research utilised grounded theory methodology, sampling occurred on the basis of gathering data about concepts, incidents and the strategies used by mothers, not numbers of 'persons' per se (Strauss & Corbin, 1990). Therefore the aim of sampling in a grounded theory study is to conduct theoretical sampling, or to collect information-rich cases until we fill gaps and refine ideas, not necessarily increase the size or numbers of the original sample (Charmaz, 2000, p. 519). Strauss and Corbin (1990, p. 177) asserted that theoretical sampling occurs on the basis that the concepts collected are deemed significant because:

1. They are repeatedly present or notably absent when comparing incident after incident, and
2. After a process of open coding they may be readily classified into relevant categories.

To access the data, the author used purposeful sampling whereby mothers were invited to participate, allowing access to information-rich cases to illuminate the phenomena under investigation. As it was a qualitative study, individuals were selected to participate in the research based on their first-hand experience with the coping phenomenon (Streubert, 1995, p. 23).

Sampling took place until 'saturation' occurred, that is, no new concepts arose. The logic and power of purposeful sampling lies in selecting information-rich cases for in-depth study. There is no need to randomly select individuals because manipulation and control is not the intent of the inquiry. The concern of the author is to develop a rich or dense description of the culture or phenomenon, rather than using sampling techniques which support generalizability of the findings.

Five mothers of babies and young children 0–5 years were accessed from long day care centres, pram walking and mothers' groups. The snowballing technique, or referral method, was used to opportunistically engage a further four mothers in a focus group discussion (Patton, 1990, p. 179). The mean age of the mothers was 34.2 years. All women described their living arrangements as married and working full-time at home. The mean number of children was 2, with mean age 21.5 months or 1¾ years.

Mothers were invited to participate in interviews at a convenient time and location. Informants had to meet the following criteria:

- mothers of one or more children within this age bracket,
- identified themselves (subjectively) as feeling well,
- living in the Pittwater area of Sydney, Australia, and
- English speaking.

This was for the purpose of being able to describe the relevant phenomena under investigation.

As all mothers were of Anglo-Saxon background, it is an assumption of this research that all mothers were aware of the dominant ideology surrounding mother-hood. That is, a 'good' mother needs to be endlessly and selflessly, emotionally and physically available to her family members at all times (Green, Hebron, & Woodward 1990; Harris, 1998; Wearing, 1984, 1996). The dominant ideology manifests itself in the way mothers experience guilt associated with their role and in their limited access to leisure, as described in works such as Harris (1998) and Green, Hebron, and Woodward (1990, pp. 118–119). The following section introduces the infor-mants who took part in the in-depth interviews. Pseudonyms are used as all names and identifiers were changed to protect the informants' confidentiality.

2.2 Introducing the Mothers

2.2.1 Wendy

Wendy is 28 years old, and has been married for 5 years. Wendy has twin boys aged 6 months. She has lived all her life in the Pittwater area of Sydney. Wendy has postgraduate qualifications in Education, and worked full-time as a Primary school teacher for approximately 4 years before becoming a full-time mother at home.

A typical day for Wendy includes getting up at 6 a.m. with the twins, and cooking, cleaning, or gardening for the rest of the day. Wendy is able to attend aqua-aerobic classes and Bible Study group once a week, while her sister minds the babies. She loves to read if she can find an opportunity. Wendy also gains excellent support from her mother, as she visits every weekday afternoon at 4 p.m. to help with the babies' feeding and bathing routine.

2.2.2 *Cynthia*

Cynthia is 32 years old, married with two daughters, aged 16 months and 3½ years. Cynthia told me of her early rises at 5.30 a.m., when her younger baby wakes, and then having to divide her time carefully with her other daughter when she wakes up. After breakfast at about 6.30 a.m., the children watch television at about 7 a.m. while Cynthia tidies up the house and puts on a load of washing. At around 9 a.m., Cynthia and the girls head out to drop off her elder daughter at pre-school, who often cries and experiences separation anxiety. Every Tuesday morning, Cynthia leads a Women's Bible Study group at her home, so will hurry home, to "frantically try to tidy up and get refreshments ready". The daytime is usually a mix of playtime with the children, visiting, shopping, and of course, housework, "So there are nappies to change, telephone calls to take and make, washing to hang out and bring in, cleaning to do".

Cynthia has to cope for prolonged periods of time without her husband, as he works for up to 6 weeks at a time at sea. Cynthia said that during those times, she has to:

> …fight a type of loneliness and a sense that time is passing so slowly and fear that I am not the most positive parent; I need to be more present, living in the moment, just be grateful.

Cynthia also talked about the adjustments that needed to be made when her husband returned to the household full-time. From being sole disciplinarian and organiser, she now had what she described as a full-time helper available, and could now afford to take a 10 min break for a shower, for instance. On the other hand, she also felt that the new situation required a degree of adjustment. Cynthia stated that her discipline style is strict, while her husband's is more laissez faire. However, when her husband was about to leave for another work period, Cynthia began to experience the dread of separation from him again.

Afternoons meant picking up Natasha from pre-school, and heading off to the park or the library. Then a routine, so typically described by all the mothers, follows of dinner, bath and bedtime. Cynthia seems to judge herself harshly, as she described herself collapsing into bed feeling very tired, but nonetheless not satisfied she had achieved much that day:

> I am happy to go to bed at the same time each night: quite exhausted, yet feeling like I have accomplished little.

2.2.3 *Vanessa*

Vanessa is a 39 year old mother of two boys, ages 3, and five months. Prior to starting a family, Vanessa worked full-time as a computer analyst programmer. She told me that she planned to return to work at some stage in the future, most probably part-time in a year or two.

Immediately after our first interview, Vanessa gave birth to her second son. Vanessa emigrated to Australia from England 12 years ago after first visiting Australia on a working visa. Vanessa's family live in England, and her husband's family is Australian and all live in New South Wales.

Vanessa tries to keep fit by attending circuit classes at the gym 3 or 4 times a week. She mentioned how she tries to fit in walking, although this can prove difficult, with two children and only a single stroller. Her walks are restricted to places, distances and speeds that her 3 year old can cope with. If Vanessa "gets a spare 5 min", as she puts it, she likes to read a book. She also enjoys occasional visits to the movies with friends, or going out to dinner with the whole family on Saturday nights:

> Our three year old likes to eat out, he'll usually sit still long enough to have a quick meal! The baby is very good so far, and is happy just to watch or sleep.

A typical day for Vanessa starts at around 5.40 a.m. if she is attending the gym. Her husband will look after her children at that time. Otherwise, children permitting, she mentioned that she likes to sleep in until 7 a.m. if possible. Vanessa described her mornings as hectic, with a routine involving making breakfasts, preparing lunches and snacks, and breastfeeding the baby. She then aims to do a load of washing and complete a few more chores around the house before heading out.

Most mornings Vanessa heads out of the house with her two children to the shops, playgroup, mothers' group, an indoor play centre or outdoor playground. Vanessa seemed to be quite pleased with the temperament of her new baby, whom she described as enjoying being out and about:

> The baby is very good and likes to be out and tries hard to stay awake to take in everything that is going on around him. My older son loves to be outside when possible. He likes going to the shops too, though I'm not so keen on taking him as he has a tendency to run off!

After arriving home around lunchtime or early afternoon, Vanessa and the children have something to eat. Then the baby will usually have a long sleep so that Vanessa can do more housework and spend some time playing with her 3 year old. Later in the afternoon, Vanessa baths the children and cooks dinner. Her family all eat together. After dinner, Vanessa plays with her children while her husband washes the dishes. Vanessa reads to her 3 year old between 7.30 pm and 8 o'clock every night. She relaxes afterwards with either a book or by watching TV:

> I give the baby his last feed for the day before going to bed between about 9.30 and 10.30 pm, hoping that the baby won't wake too many times in the night! He occasionally sleeps through till 7 am, but usually wakes around 3 or 4 am for a feed and on a bad night he wakes 3 or 4 times! Thankfully these times don't happen too often.

2.2.4 Trish

Trish is 35 years old and has lived in this same geographic location all her life. Her interests include sailing, art and the outdoors. She is the mother of a 2¾ year old daughter and 8 month old son. She described herself as "fairly organised, caring and fairly level-headed". Before becoming a mother, Trish worked as a Personal Assistant to the Vice President of a large global insurance company.

Trish described warmly how she and the two children sit in bed and read stories after they wake between 5 and 6 a.m. They have usually had breakfast and are all dressed by 8.30 a.m. On a typical day, Trish would try to do a little housework, and then when the baby was asleep, spend some time with her older child. Similar to other mothers' stories, when the baby wakes, they usually head out to go shopping, to the park, visiting friends, playgroup or mothers' group.

Home around 2 p.m., the baby would normally have another sleep while Trish played with her older child in the back yard, and sometimes completed a few more chores. The children would have dinner at the relatively early time of 4.30 p.m., and the baby is bathed and in bed by 6 p.m. Her older child is bathed and in bed just before Trish has dinner with her husband at about 7.30 p.m. Trish leads a very organised lifestyle. She often emphasised the importance of planning and organisation. Paradoxically, she told me that in general, "there is little time" for herself. She will often head to bed by 9.30 p.m. as she is still involved in night-time breastfeeding.

2.2.5 Sarah

Sarah is a vivacious 37 year old, married with 2 children, aged 4 months, and 5 years. Sarah worked as an Office Manager prior to having children and now works full-time at home. Sarah is very talented at interior design and her home reflected this sense of planned colour and style. She and her husband also made a living out of property development whereby they purchased blocks of land or older houses, and spent a period of time renovating or re-building, then selling for a profit. Sarah described this as having been profitable for the couple previously, but with the addition of children, the process of project management was made that much more difficult.

Sarah was very attuned to the importance of her social network, and valued highly the opportunity to go on regular outings with 'the girls'. Sarah stated she was currently well, however 5 years ago had experienced postnatal depression following the birth of her first child, with subsequent marriage problems, and eventual reconciliation.

2.3 Conceptual Framework

The research began with the area of coping strategies used by mothers of young children, and then allowed the theory to emerge from the data. The theory arose from a set of well-developed categories (e.g. themes, concepts) that were systematically inter-related through statements of relationship to form a theoretical framework that helped to explain the coping phenomena in this context (Strauss & Corbin, 1998, p. 22). From capturing, fracturing and closely analysing the data, the main themes emerged. The aim of grounded theory research is to build rather than test theory. The author needed to complete a certain amount of general pre-reading to increase her theoretical sensitivity and awareness of the area. However, she did not enter the research with any pre-conceived theoretical models to explain the phenomena.

Therefore, as the mothers felt they had developed an effective coping strategy, they felt a sense of increased confidence and control over their own situation. The increased sense of control led to greater feelings of subjective well-being. Health promotion includes increasing one's control over one's health. What did emerge as the research progressed was that self-empowerment includes having sets of skills or practices enabling the individual to believe she/he exerts some sort of control over one's environment (Tones, 1993, p. 7).

2.4 Indicators and Instruments

The indicators present in the qualitative data were derived from the women's own responses. The author developed theories grounded in the informant's experience of social reality. Otherwise she could construct and impose a fictional view of the informants' reality. According to Minichiello, Aroni, Timewell, and Alexander (1992), indicators revealing people's experiences of their own social reality must be based on their routinely constructed interpretations.

The informants' own expressions of coping experiences were used to indicate examples of perceived coping or to describe strategies. Grounded theory methodology is designed to guide researchers in producing theory that is "conceptually dense"—that is, with many conceptual relationships (Strauss & Corbin, 1994, p. 278). Secondly, grounded theories are always traceable to the data that gave rise to them. Therefore the mothers' own terminology and descriptions provide the most accurate account of the phenomena under examination. For an accurate account or reflection of people's reality, personal documentations are needed. Reinharz (1992, p. 18) describes statements from the women themselves as most representative of "...the handwoven fabric of their daily work and lives".

To better understand the nature of the coping process, Lazarus (1999), co-founder of the original "Ways of Coping Questionnaire", now recommends in-depth interviewing. Therefore, for *Managing Motherhood*, the indicators of perceived effective to ineffective coping were obtained from the qualitative interview transcripts. This included the mothers' claims and expressions. Typical expressions taken to be indicative of effective to ineffective coping (Lazarus, 1999, p. 152) during the research included:

- Improved ability to cope—Includes expressions of self-empowerment or self-appraisals of improvements in coping. For example, "I cope much better now" or "My coping skills are better now, I've discovered I can now manage that stressor more constructively than I used to".

- Efficacious coping outcomes—Reflected in self-appraisals of successful coping outcomes. Includes typical statements, "I've found this is the best thing to do", or "Yes, that worked well".
- Non-efficacious coping outcomes—Are self-appraisals of unsuccessful coping outcomes, such as "That's not doing any good".

An instrument or Interview Focus Schedule was developed to help focus the conversations with informants about their coping experiences. Following the initial interview, an 'Issues Paper' was developed outlining the findings as summarised from the grounded theory analysis. This was shown to the mothers prior to the second interview as a form of validating or checking the accuracy of the data. The informants were asked if they wished to clarify, change or refute any of the issues raised previously, or if they had anything else to add. In what Crotty (1998, p. 83) describes as "intuiting the data", the informants themselves were invited to peruse the data, to support and validate the claim that the themes they pointed to were genuinely able to be found in the data.

The procedures involved in the collection of the data will now be examined.

2.5   Data Collection

In-depth, semi-structured or focused interviews (hereafter, 'in-depth' interviews) were used as the means of gaining understanding of the informant's lived experience of coping and implementing strategies. In-depth interviews, with minimal researcher interference, were selected because:

- the researcher did not wish to enter the interviews with pre-conceived ideas about content outcomes
- the interviews were organised only around an area of particular interest and what was of importance to the informants was allowed to emerge (May, 1991, p. 191).

That is, there was a phenomena of interest, and while a large degree of leeway was allowed for the conversation to be informant-driven, the author kept in mind the need to remain focused or within topical limits.

Minichiello, Aroni, Timewell, and Alexander (1995) argued that the term 'between researcher and informant' illustrates the egalitarian relation of power and roles in the interview. The mothers were labelled as 'informants' due to the highly valued, relevant and informative nature of their views and opinions. Further, "use of the term informants illustrates the position that qualitative researchers ascribe to" (Streubert, 1995, p. 23). In-depth interviews are most likely to lead to greatest rapport, understanding and balance of power between researcher and informant (Minichiello, Aroni, Timewell, & Alexander 1995).

Another benefit of in-depth or open-ended interviews, as argued by Patton (1990, p. 46), is that what is meaningful may be represented and told by the mothers themselves, without pigeon-holing their responses into standardised categories. A conversational method was employed, which according to Minichiello et al. (1995) is more likely to reveal issues most important to the informant, as expressed in their own words. By not approaching the interview with a totally pre-determined set of sequenced or close-ended questions, the informants themselves could set the research boundaries in terms of the research question.

Following institutional ethics approval, the informants took part in a series of two in-depth interviews. The first interview aimed to open up general discussion around the topic of coping and coping strategies. It aimed to discover what was important, as raised by the mothers. A focus schedule assisted the author in 're-focusing' the topic, and prevented the conversation moving greatly away from the topic of coping strategies. The Issues Paper also helped to funnel discussion for the second interview, helping focus on relating the experiences and attitudes that were relevant to the problem (Burgess, 1982, p. 107).

In what Patton (1990) describes as opportunistic sampling, and typical in a grounded theory study, an opportunity arose during data collection to conduct a focus group as another means of accessing the opinions and ideas of a similar group of mothers. Opportunistic sampling takes advantage of any new opportunities arising during data collection. The opportunity consisted of a snowballing technique, whereby Sarah invited the author to attend a Play Group session during morning tea, where she had arranged for a small group of four of her friends, who also had children 0–5 years and lived locally, to take part in a group interview. Using the principles outlined by Kitzinger (1997), a focus group interview was conducted. The focus group method used for this research was appropriate, as the participants had perused the same Issues Paper beforehand, and the author encouraged them to explore any issues raised, or generate their own questions and pursue their own priorities. The group processes can help to explore and clarify views in ways that would be less easily accessible in a one to one interview Kitzinger (1997, p. 37). The reflection process undertaken by focus group participants in response to the author's questions [or Issues Paper], gives rise synergistically to insights and solutions that would not have otherwise come about. "They [focus groups] can be used to both supplement and validate other qualitative techniques" (Baum 1999, p. 160).

Using a small group of four mothers was preferable when the participants had intense related experiences and a great deal to share about the topic [as mothers]. The downside is that group dynamics, peer pressure or strong views by a particular individual may have dominated or inhibited an individual from airing a dissenting view. The other disadvantage is that responses are not independent or individualised. The benefit of focus groups is that it is a timely and economical method of possibly being alerted to what is considered significant within the area under focus (Minichiello et al., 1995, p. 65).

The use of this additional data collection method can be referred to as triangulation. Further, by showing the informants in the main part of the research, and the focus group participants, the 'Issues Paper', the author conducted a stakeholder check. Thomas (2000, p. 19) referred to this as the process of taking the draft findings to people such as research participants, service providers and any others who have an interest. The author was able to seek comment on the extent to which the findings were consistent with the mothers' everyday experiences, and whether the findings assisted understanding of the topic being investigated.

All interviews were audio-taped and fully transcribed verbatim using a word processing package. All transcript material was used for data analysis purposes. As analysis of the data is completed continually and immediately after each stage of data collection, data collection continued until theoretical saturation took place. That is, until no new data were being unearthed from the interviews (Strauss & Corbin, 1998, p. 292). The methods used for the book to analyse the data collected will now be examined.

2.6   Data Analysis

After the interview data were transcribed, a content analysis was employed to discover the major categories or themes to emerge characterising the strategies mothers used to cope. A grounded theory approach allowed what was important to the phenomena of coping strategies to emerge from the interview data collected and transcribed (Strauss & Corbin, 1990).

The four key steps involved in the systematic techniques and procedures of grounded theory analysis as described by Strauss and Corbin (1990) are:

1. *Coding or analysing the data*. Open coding involved fracturing or breaking down the data. Line by line, sentence by sentence, the data were examined, compared, and identified or conceptualised. Conceptual labels were placed on discrete happenings, events and phenomena. The author made constant comparisons and asked questions about the data. Coding ceased at the point of theoretical saturation when no additional or new concepts continued to emerge. These comparisons and analyses of the data informed the author of a saturation point where further interviewing could cease.
2. *Classifying or grouping these concepts into meaningful categories*. A category was formed by classifying similar or related concepts together under a higher or more abstract theme or label. The characteristics and properties of the categories were noted.
3. *Axial coding*. This procedure involved making connections between a category and its sub-categories or concepts, and proposing and analysing links between categories.
4. *Developing possible theories*. The final step required examination of the major themes to emerge. Theoretical explanations could then be systematically developed.

According to Charmaz (2000, p. 520), as we define our categories as saturated, we begin the process of rewriting our memos or analysis in expanded, more analytic form. This whole process was aided by what Strauss and Corbin (1990, p. 41) call "theoretical sensitivity". Personal qualities such as insight or experience can aid the author in being able to detect or be aware of any subtleties of meaning in the data

(Glaser & Strauss, 1967). In terms of theoretical sensitivity, the author has gained certain insights and knowledge in understanding the informants due to her experience as a mother of two children. She has a long-term background in health promotion research into the 'coping experience'.

2.7 Conclusion

A search of the literature reveals that little past research has been undertaken into mothers' coping strategies from their own perspectives. This is especially so for mothers who identify as well. The author was interested in exploring all of these things, and finding out about the lived experiences of a group of 'real' mothers. Therefore an in-depth qualitative research study was undertaken and this book presents insights into a new wellness perspective of coping. Such qualitative approaches are to be recommended as they value the subjective experiences of women.

The qualitative methods used to obtain the key data reported in *Managing Motherhood* align themselves more to offering opportunities for obtaining individual responses. In this way we are able to ascertain what it means to the mothers to cope, and report on their experiences in their own words. *Managing Motherhood* is underpinned by a new, health-promoting definition of coping. The subjective perceptions and expressions of one's own experiences are valued and paramount to understanding the phenomena of coping. The next section introduces the informants featured in the book.

Chapter 3 provides a review of the related research literature to gain an understanding of research published to date in the area of mothers' coping strategies.

References

Baum, F. (1999). *The new public health: An Australian perspective*. Melbourne: Oxford University Press.

Burgess, R. G. (1982). *Field research: Sourcebook and field manual*. London: Allen & Unwin.

Carpenter, D. R. (1995). Grounded theory research approach. In H. J. Streubert & D. R. Carpenter (Eds.), *Qualitative research in nursing. Advancing the humanistic* imperative (pp. 145–61). Philadelphia: J. B. Lippincott.

Charmaz, K. (2000). Grounded theory: Objectivist and constructivist methods. In N. K. Denzin & Y. S. Lincoln (Eds.), *Handbook of Qualitative Research* (2nd ed., pp. 509–536). Thousand Oaks: Sage.

Chenitz, W. C., & Swanson, J. M. (1986). Qualitative research using grounded theory. In W. C. Chenitz & J. M. Swanson (Eds.), *From practice to grounded theory. Qualitative research in nursing* (pp. 3–15). Menlo Park, CA: Addison-Wesley.

Crotty, M. (1998). *The foundations of social research. Meaning and perspective in the research process* Crows Nest, Sydney: Allen and Unwin.

Glaser, B. G., & Strauss, A. L. (1967). *Discovery of Grounded Theory: Strategies for qualitative research*. Chicago: Aldine.

Green, E., Hebron, S., & Woodward, D. (1990). *Women's Leisure, What Leisure?*. London: Macmillan Education.

Harris, N. (1998). Coping with young children: how do mothers do it? In *Proceedings of the 6th Australian Institute of Family Studies (AIFS) Conference* (pp. 1–5). Melbourne: AIFS.

Kitzinger, J. (1997). Introducing focus groups. In N. Mays & C. Pope (Eds.), *Qualitative research in health care* (pp. 36–44). London: British Medical Journal Publications.

Lazarus, R. S. (1999). *Stress and emotion: A new synthesis*. New York: Springer.

May, K. A. (1991). Interview techniques in qualitative research: Concerns and challenges. In J. M. Morse (Ed.), *Qualitative nursing research. A contemporary dialogue* (pp. 188–201). Newbury Park, CA: Sage.

Minichiello, V., Aroni, R., Timewell, E., & Alexander, L. (1992). *In-depth interviewing* (1st ed.). Melbourne: Longman.

Minichiello, V., Aroni, R., Timewell, E., & Alexander, L. (1995). *In-depth interviewing* (2nd ed.). Melbourne: Longman.

Minichiello, V., Fulton, G., & Sullivan, G. (1999). Posing qualitative research questions. In V. Minichiello, G. Fulton, G. Sullivan, & R. Axford (Eds.), *Handbook for research methods in health sciences* (pp. 35–56). Sydney: Addison-Wesley.

Patton, M. (1990). *Qualitative evaluation and research methods* (2nd ed.). Newbury Park USA: Sage.

Punch, K. F. (1998). *Introduction to social research. Quantitative and qualitative approaches*. London: Sage.

Reinharz, S. (1992). *Feminist methods in social research*. New York: Oxford University Press.

Strauss, A., & Corbin, J. (1990). *Basics of qualitative research. Grounded theory procedures and techniques*. Newbury Park, CA: Sage.

Strauss, A., & Corbin, J. (1994). Grounded theory methodology. An overview. In N. K. Denzin & Y. S. Lincoln (Eds.), *Handbook of qualitative research* (1st ed., pp. 273–85). Thousand Oaks, CA: Sage.

Strauss, A., & Corbin, J. (1998). *Basics of qualitative research. Grounded theory procedures and techniques* (2nd ed.). Thousand Oaks, CA: Sage.

Streubert, H. J. (1995). What is nursing knowledge? In H. J. Streubert & D. R. Carpenter (Eds.), *Qualitative research in nursing. Advancing the humanistic imperative* (pp. 15–28). Philadelphia: J. B. Lippincott.

Thomas, D. R. (2000). Qualitative evidence: The contribution of qualitative research to evidence-based medicine. *HRC Newsletter, 34,* 18–19.

Tones, K. (1993). The theory of health promotion: Implications for nursing. In J. Wilson-Barnett & J. Macleod-Clark (Eds.), *Research in health promotion and nursing* (pp. 3–14). Houndmills, UK: Macmillan.

Wearing, B. (1984). *The ideology of motherhood*. Sydney: George Allen and Unwin.

Wearing, B. (1996). *Gender: The pain and the pleasure of difference*. Melbourne: Longman.

Chapter 3
Managing Motherhood

Abstract Coping includes individual efforts to manage stressors and maintain feelings of well-being. During early motherhood, women are faced with many stressors and often crave time-out, space and sleep. However, when they take timeout, they are also likely to experience guilt or find it difficult to ask for help. 'What it means' for mothers who identify as well *to* be coping has not been researched previously in-depth. The focus has also been on 'not coping', the problems that exist, and on marginalised and unwell groups. To achieve healthy coping, women may need to relax their expectations slightly, and focus on their own wellness, versus attempting to attain perfection.

3.1 Introduction

The notion of coping derives from the Darwinian concept of human evolution or adaptation to the environment (Tudor, 1999). Together with self-esteem, an ability to maintain healthy relationships and effective decision-making, the capacity for effective coping is a key element of mental health. A sense of coping with challenges positively influences our perception of well-being, self-worth and self-esteem. If we feel in control of our life and environment, we experience a greater sense of empowerment and well-being. Managing motherhood and gaining a sense of coping provides women with greater quality of life satisfaction (Bowling, 1997, p. 9).

Coping includes any individual efforts are subjectively evaluated as dealing constructively with daily stressors. This results in a greater sense of empowerment or control. However, for many mothers, the period of coping with a new child can represent a period of great stress and change (Walker & Wilging, 2000). Some mothers are so seriously affected by the disruption and stress that they develop emotional disorders after the birth (Currie & Develin, 1999). As early motherhood is viewed as demanding and stressful (Currie, 2008; Michelson, 1985; Walker & Wilging, 2000; Wearing, 1990), researching the ways mothers have attempted to successfully deal

© The Author(s) 2018
J. L. Currie, *Managing Motherhood*, SpringerBriefs in Well-Being and Quality
of Life Research, https://doi.org/10.1007/978-981-13-0338-8_3

with perceived stressors is appropriate. This chapter reviews the related research literature on coping strategies used by mothers of young children.

3.2 Mothers of Young Children: What Do They Cope with?

While many women experience great joy at becoming a mother, many women also express a loss of freedom and autonomy (Currie, 2004). Mothers often feel anxious or tense from the amount of caring involved, combined with lack of sleep, and space or time to themselves (Sethi, 1995). Sethi's (1995) study identified an emotional crisis many new mothers experience while coping with the first 6 months after birth (see Table 3.1). However, she did not reveal how mothers cope with day-to-day stressors in any detail.

Guilt is another major emotional issue that mothers have to cope with. A mother often feels that she needs to 'be there' for her child all of the time and feels guilty when not available (Littlewood & McHugh, 1997, p. 75). She also feels guilt if she's not enjoying herself, not performing at top levels or feeling positive emotions in response to being a new mother. The ideology of motherhood can also pressure women into denying they're even experiencing any negative feelings or reactions (Crouch & Manderson, 1993, p. 159).

Many mothers also have to singularly cope with feelings of stress or dissatisfaction with the childcare experience, and this has changed little over the past 30 years (Boulton, 1983; Littlewood & McHugh, 1997; Maushart, 1997; Oakley, 1979). For example, Littlewood and McHugh (1997, pp. 75–76) discovered that 66% of a sample of middle class and 44% of a sample of working class mothers found looking after children full-time to be an irritating and unrewarding experience due to:

- Increased levels of stress associated with having sole responsibility for young children and being available 'on demand'.
- Lack of time to one's self.
- Resulting loss of self-identity and individuality associated with becoming a mother.

Table 3.1 Sources of stress experienced in the first 6 months of motherhood (Sethi, 1995, p. 239)

The dialectic of tensions existing within the new mother between…		
Love for the baby	⇔	Willing to give to herself
Attending to baby promptly	⇔	Feeling lonely and confined
Being flexible and patient	⇔	Feeling afraid, frustrated
Feeling challenged	⇔	Loss of autonomy, freedom and predictability
Adapting to change	⇔	Re-evaluating—who am I?
New identity and transformation	⇔	Ambivalent feelings and loss of previous independence

Mercer's (1995) study noted how mothers were often stressed by lack of time to self and constant responsibility. She concluded, "Mothers had no time to read or take an outing; they felt tied down and isolated" (Mercer, 1995, p. 117). The stress associated with parenting and daily lifestyles of new mothers combined with diminished social support may intensify emotional distress and depressed mood of new mothers (Beck, 1996; O'Hara, Schlechte, Lewis, & Varner, 1995). If women are not able to cope with stressful demands of major lifestyle changes, they may become susceptible to health problems in the first postpartum year (Lenz, Parks, Jenkins, & Jarrett, 1986).

A longitudinal study of mothers' parenting stress over the first 3 years of the infant's life carried out by (Mulsow, Caldera, Pursley, Reifman, & Huston, 2002) found that a mother's own personality was the most predictive factor of a woman's degree of parenting stress. That is, women with a more relaxed or positive outlook in their general nature tended to be more resistant to stress. Other factors noted as most positively impacting on mother's stress levels included intimacy with partner (at 0–6 months and during the third year), general social support (during the second year), and child's temperament (at 1 month and 3 years of age of the child). Social isolation, loneliness and lack of support are sources of stress that can negatively affect coping. When mothers are well supported by family, friends or colleagues, they often cope more effectively (Crouch & Manderson, 1993).

Mothers also need to feel they have adequate time to be able to deal with competing demands. Mothers with multiple tasks or roles to perform experience greater time pressures and are at risk of role overload (Crouch & Manderson, 1993; Raskin, Kummel, & Bannister, 1998). There is a paucity of research investigating factors contributing to mothers' fatigue, such as sleep deficits, tension or anxiety.

One factor that does impact greatly on a mother's mental health is body image and physical appearance (Currie & Develin, 1999). Women's bodies undergo immense changes in weight and appearance pre- and post-birth. Ninety-five percent of mothers admit to coping with feelings of being unattractive and overweight (Mercer, 1995). Approximately half (21/37) of the respondents (average age 32 years with 1 child, 12 months old) in the study by Currie (1999, p. 178) were dissatisfied with their body image, commonly stating "I feel overweight", "I need to lose weight", or "I don't like my postnatal shape". Concerns about body shape most commonly include having a flabby abdomen and wishing to regain one's earlier, pre-pregnant shape.

If a mother feels depressed, this can also impact on her mental health through feelings of guilt, being overwhelmed, or a sense of inadequacy through not coping (Mercer, 1995). Mental health will be improved if a mother feels like she is coping with everyday tasks and incorporating the parent role into her identity (Mercer, 1995). It doesn't help when tasks completed by mothers such as housework or childcare remain unpaid and undervalued by society, only noticed when *not* completed.

It has been established that motherhood is stressful and requires employment of plenty of coping strategies to deal with unpredictable circumstances (Crouch & Manderson, 1993; Dix, 1987). Further, "It is incumbent on the women themselves to resolve these problems and cope" (Crouch & Manderson, 1993, p. 161). The adaptation or coping process women use to manage motherhood is little understood (Currie, 2009; Sethi, 1995). It would help new mothers build resilience if they could be informed of helpful strategies, as Sethi (1995, p. 243) says, "to master the art of motherhood". Unfortunately the implications of much of the media and literature portraying perfection in the art of mothering mean that a mother may experience outside societal pressures to perform well in her attempt to be a 'good' mother (Welles-Nystrom, New, & Richman, 1994).

3.3   Coping with the 'Art of Motherhood'

Is there an 'art' to motherhood? An art, which if mastered, means the woman attains the status of 'good' mother? Who judges this status? The mother herself? Or does day-to-day mothering rather involve a series of down-to-earth tasks and events that need to be coped with so that a mother feels subjectively in control? If there is an 'art' to motherhood, it has not been realistically documented, nor effectively in the mothers' own voices, until this book. It should only matter if a mother herself feels like she is coping. There is a general lack of research available on the importance for individual mothers to free themselves from ideological pressures of trying to meet the 'successful ideal'.

Oakley (1979) argued that women often felt lost or disappointed when they believed they had not attained the culturally valued, idealised and romanticised vision of motherhood. Mothers may feel frustration, tiredness, sorrow and constraint at times in response to the more mundane or thankless aspects of their lifestyle, in addition to experiencing positive feelings of self-worth, happiness rewards and satisfaction (Littlewood & McHugh, 1997). New mothers are expected by society to be coping and even feel fulfilled from the experience. For those mothers who personally feel tense, angry, resentful, frightened, trapped or simply overwhelmingly sad, these emotions can be a source of puzzlement and internal shame (Crouch & Manderson, 1993, p. 160).

Maushart (1997) purported that social pressures resulted in some mothers even 'faking' it and pretending that they were enjoying themselves even when they were not coping or were actually feeling depressed. While it is often expected that the events mothers have to cope with are fairly standard (Sethi, 1995), each mother's experiences are unique and have not been adequately investigated previously (Maushart, 1997; Phoenix, Woollett, & Lloyd, 1991). It is no wonder mothers are often overwhelmed and stressed with their roles, because there is a lack of preparation for motherhood and a lack of realistic guidelines available outlining how to cope (Crouch & Manderson, 1993; Littlewood & McHugh, 1997). Most attention is directed towards surviving pregnancy and labour; relatively short-term events. However, Crouch and Manderson (1993, p. 135) described caring for the new baby as totally different. It is continuous, ever-present, and mothers need to cope with demanding and unpredictable circumstances as they arise (Crouch & Manderson, 1993, p. 135).

With the changing role of fatherhood and partners, an area barely mentioned in the literature is their contribution in parenting, and in turn, assisting mothers to cope (Carpenter, 2002). Prokos (2003) revealed results of interviews with fathers who revealed hopes to re-shape dominant ideologies about the roles of fathers and mothers into a more neutral idea of parenting. However, their underlying beliefs were nevertheless stereotypical and not reflective of true gender equality.

Milkie, Bianchi, Mattingly, and Robinson (2002) stated that recent cultural expectations about fathers' involvement in childrearing may have changed more rapidly than fathers' actual behaviours in the home, creating what Milkie, Bianchi, Mattingly, & Robinson (2002, p. 37) described as, "discrepancies between parenting ideals and realities that can generate tensions in family life". For example, in their study, less than ideal father o partner involvement in disciplining children was associated with mothers' higher stress levels. Discrepancies in mothers' expectations of, to actual fatherly involvement in play and monitoring children, was correlated with mothers' increased feelings of unfairness in the household division of labour.

The bulk of the literature on mothers and coping shows that mothers either willingly or unwillingly take on the bulk of the family nurturing and caring. To help mothers cope more effectively, husbands and partners may need to increase involvement in childrearing and be educated about what mothers feel are equitable contributory levels. Discrepancies were revealed in the literature between mothers and fathers to fathers' ideal and actual parenting involvement levels.

Research into detailing the strategies mothers use in order to cope is needed in order to more fully understand their overall lifestyle and methods of coping. The following section identifies some of the practical ways that women deal with the mothering role, as reported in the research literature.

3.4 What Strategies Help Mothers Cope?

According to Musil and Abraham (1986), coping is the effort required to deal with a difficult experience. If coping includes individual efforts aimed at controlling one's experiences, then successful coping will lead to greater feelings of individual or internal locus of control. The research literature often characterises motherhood as a constant struggle involving loss of control over one's personal space and time (Wearing, 1990). For mothers, effective coping may therefore mean feeling in control of one's tasks and gaining freedom through access to a space of one's own (Currie, 2004; Wearing, 1990). Increased feelings of effective coping will help a mother feel in harmony with her role, and be more relaxed, with "a sense of comfort about where she has been and where she is going" (Mercer, 1995, p. 13).

A mother may cope more effectively if she tunes into her own needs and doesn't keep up "a stoic façade of 'I'm coping', because that's what good mothers do" (Dix, 1987, p. 201). Being able to accept outside help readily without feeling guilty may also assist coping. According to Dix (1987, pp. 201–202), it is healthy for a mother to develop a conscious awareness of her own needs, rather than always worrying about the baby. She recommends that a mother focuses on herself more, on what the stress is doing to her, rather than always worrying about its effect on the baby. To achieve greater wellbeing, Dix (1987) also advises women to not deny her own needs or see herself as unimportant. That kind of attitude can lead to PND, because we are at greater risk of not meeting our own basic needs, and can lose our own sense of identity and self-esteem. Achieving guilt-free 'time out' from the motherhood role can be a valuable way for women to reduce stress and pursue interests to potentially raise self-esteem (Currie, 2004, 2018). One method a mother can use to focus on her own needs is to access leisure. Leisure provides us with coping factors, including perceived freedom, intrinsic motivation (not boredom), internality or internal locus of control, hardiness, enjoyment, skill, distraction and social support. Therefore, leisure can potentially assist mothers to cope by buffering daily stressors (Currie, 2004, 2018).

Activities like leisure or exercise undertaken in the postpartum period are important for women to prioritise as (a) they have the potential to improve women's immediate health and well-being (Currie, 2004; Koltyn & Schultes, 1997; Sampselle, Seng, Yeo, Killion, & Oakley, 1999; Walker & Wilging, 2000); and (b) women normally tend to abandon or reduce participation in these activities at this critical phase of the lifespan (Currie & Develin, 1999; Tulman, Fawcett, Groblewski, & Silverman, 1990). Physical activity has the potential to improve mothers' body image. All but a few (32/37) of the mothers participating in a pramwalking program believed that it made them feel more positively about their own body shape and would recommend it to others (Currie, 1999).

Wearing (1990) interviewed 60 mothers of first babies 1–8 months old (30 working class, 30 middle-class) and found that a strong relationship existed between time spent by the mother on her own leisure or creating her own space, and aspects of mental and general health. Wearing (1990) described a woman's transition to motherhood as a crisis in terms of decreased time and space to self, due mainly to a mother's almost total responsibility for childcare. She discovered that leisure helped mothers cope with these limitations and increases in positive leisure experiences were able to reduce tension, stress and improve health indices. "Leisure is the free choice to do something or nothing for your own enjoyment" (Wearing, 1990, p. 5). Seventy seven percent of participants believed they have a right to some time and space for themselves at least once a week, and 90% felt that leisure was important. However, it was discovered that to access leisure, women needed to make an effort themselves to make this space and it required forward planning and organisation. Women also needed to juggle with the guilt experienced when exerting the right to take time-out. Further, it was also concluded that a father's assistance was needed: a shared approach to parenting.

It is now thought by government policymakers that parenting programs have an important role to play in the improvement of maternal health (Barlow & Cohen, 2003). Studies by Mullin, Quigley and Glanville (1994), Scott and Stradling (1987) and Todres and Bunston (1993) show that parenting programs can have significant positive effects on parenting attitudes and practices, marital relations, parenting stress, and maternal functioning including levels of anxiety, depression and self-esteem. These programs teach parents how to use a range of basic behavioural and cognitive strategies for managing children's behaviour (Barlow & Cohen, 2003). Most programs reported in the literature also seem to be targeted at parents of children with a wide range of problems, or disadvantage, however these factors were not assessed for their influence on outcomes. Another danger noted was that parents who drop out of such programs were often blamed for their own failure to complete the course, rather than the appropriateness of the program being called into question (Barlow & Cohen, 2003).

A recent systematic review of randomised controlled trials showed that parenting programs are effective in improving behavioural problems in young children (Barlow, 1997; Barlow & Stewart-Brown, 2000). Focus groups were conducted for a group of mothers of children with special needs after they participated in a short-term parenting-education intervention (Helitzer, Cunningham-Sabo, Van Leit, & Crowe, 2002). The mothers expressed that participating in the program helped them to feel strong, attractive, resilient, respected and accepted. Prior to taking part in the program, their self-perception included images of feeling overwhelmed with daily routines and caring, loss of identity, being socially isolated, and expecting less from their careers. After participating in the program, they expressed they had gained coping skills such as an ability to more effectively advocate for themselves and their child, more relaxed expectations about their responsibilities and what is needed to care well for their child, and increased self-care practices (Helitzer et al., 2002, p. 30).

Harris (1998) investigated the coping strategies used by five Townsville mothers of young children (0–5 years). The study was limited to studying childcare coping strategies, not miscellaneous everyday events or issues openly nominated by the mothers themselves. Three types of coping were discovered as being utilised by the mothers. These included instrumental, introspective and organisational support.

Instrumental strategies related to how the practical aspects of daily living could be accomplished, for instance using the television to relax a tired child, cooking dinner early or letting the child choose her/his own clothes. Introspective strategies referred to methods involving the examination and use of the respondent's own mental processes, thoughts, feelings and inner self as a means of coping. Examples included withdrawing from a difficult situation, telling yourself you are not on your own, accepting the chaos of parenting, and trying to maintain your own identity and personality. Organisational strategies involved arranging other people or events to assist with childcare management. Thinking ahead and organisational skills were important aspects of this category of coping. Typical scenarios included accessing the grandmother to care for a child, social networking, socialising with other families who have young children, being well organised, and asking a husband or partner for help.

However, proximity to one's own mother did not necessarily mean extra support was always available. Harris' (1998) findings contradicted the findings of Wearing (1984, 1990), who asserted that mothers were always available to assist daughters with their own families and tasks, characterising the 'good' mother relationship.

While Harris (1998) originally classified the strategies as either internal (not requiring assistance from others) or external (required assistance from other people, institutions), she then found that using a 'reciprocity filter' was more helpful. That is, she viewed strategies in terms of the likely amount of reciprocal obligation that would be incurred if the strategy was engaged. Respondents were more likely to employ strategies where their reciprocal obligations were least. The mothers followed a two-step approach in the decision-making process regarding selection of strategies: (a) firstly, could the mothers rely on herself to engage the strategy or did she need to negotiate others? The preference was to rely on self, and (b) secondly, if it was not possible to rely on one's self, then the mother assessed the nature of the relationship with the person she was going to request help from. Questions the mother would ask before accessing the help included, How equitable is the relationship? What do I need to do to equalise the relationship? Is it possible to meet this [future] obligation?

The coping strategies selected by mothers in Harris' (1998) study were consistent with an ideological context emphasising maternal responsibility. That is, the mother needed to manage her situation on her own. If she could not, then she at least needed to select coping strategies that involved the least "reciprocal obligation", or return favours to others. The finding that all respondents indicated that they, the mother, accepted primary responsibility for implementing childcare strategies is consistent with Wearing's (1990) research with 107 mothers of young children, where 90% indicated they assumed primary responsibility for the care of their baby. Fifty-six percent of the group in Wearing's (1990) study reported that they assumed this role because it was socially imposed on them by others including husbands. Only 12% assumed prime responsibility because they believed it was the woman's role.

While Harris (1998) interviewed respondents who were also her friends, she concluded that this approach was consistent with the feminist theoretical context of her study, valuing the subjective experience of women. Harris (1998) argued that if service provision in the area of helping mothers to cope is to be relevant, then the voices of people (or potential clients) in similar circumstances must be heard.

3.5 Conclusion

Positive coping strategies for mothers may relate to women having more relaxed expectations about their caring responsibilities. Only one published study by Harris (1998) recommended mothers accept the chaos of parenting. In contrast, the majority of the literature urges or contains (a) instructions on how mothers can master the 'art of motherhood', or (b) how marginalised groups deviate from the ideal.

Qualitative research using grounded theory to uncover issues as described by mothers themselves has not been conducted previously in this area. This book fills this gap in the literature. In writing *Managing Motherhood*, I have explained what coping means to real mothers, from their own perspective. I have taken a new wellness paradigm. Coping through healthy means and strategies builds self-esteem and creates an overall sense of personal competence and subjective well-being. What has not been exposed previously, is an explanation, in their own words, of how mothers themselves feel when they are coping. What does it mean in terms of their overall lifestyle to be effectively coping? Chapter 4 describes the lived experience of coping from the perspectives of a group of real mothers.

References

Barlow, J. (1997). *Systematic review of the effectiveness of parent-education programs in improving the behavior of 3–7 year old children*. Oxford, UK: Health Services Research Unit.

Barlow, J., & Cohen, E. (2003). Parent-training programs for improving maternal psychosocial health (Cochrane Review). *The Cochrane Library, Issue 1*. Oxford: Update Software.

Barlow, J., & Stewart-Brown, S. (2000). Review articles: Behavioural problems and group-based parent-education programs. *Journal of Developmental Behavior and Pediatrics, 21, 4*.

Beck, C. T. (1996). A meta-analysis of predictors of postpartum depression. *Nursing Research, 45*, 297–303.

Boulton, M. (1983). *On Being a mother*. London: Tavistock.

Bowling, A. (1997). *Measuring health: A review of quality of life measurement scales* (2nd ed.). Philadelphia: Open University Press.

Carpenter, B. (2002). Inside the portrait of the family: The importance of fatherhood. *Early Child Development & Care, 172*, 195–202.

Crouch, M., & Manderson, L. (1993). *New motherhood. Cultural and personal transitions in the 1980s*. Camberwell, VC: Gordon & Breach.

Currie, J. L. (1999). Influences on personal body image: New mothers in a pram-walking program. In *Proceedings of the Body Culture Conference. 2nd National Body Image Conference* (pp. 178–183), Melbourne.

Currie, J. L. (2004). Motherhood, stress and the exercise experience: Freedom or constraint? *Leisure Studies, 23*, 225–242.

Currie, J. L. (2008). Conditions affecting perceived coping for new mothers: Analysis of a pilot study, Sydney, Australia. *The International Journal of Mental Health Promotion, 10*, 34–41.

Currie, J. L. (2009). Managing motherhood: Strategies used by new mothers to maintain perceptions of wellness. *Health Care for Women International, 30*, 655–670.

Currie, J. L. (2018). *Radical leisure. How mothers gain well-being and control through participation in exercise classes*. Champaign, IL: Common Ground Research Networks.

Currie, J. L., & Develin, E. D. (1999). *Stroll your way to well-being*. Woolloomooloo, Sydney: Department for Women.

Dix, C. (1987). *The new mother syndrome. Coping with postnatal stress and depression*. North Sydney: Allen and Unwin.

Harris, N. (1998). Coping with young children: how do mothers do it? In *Proceedings of the 6th Australian Institute of Family Studies (AIFS) Conference* (pp. 1–5). Melbourne: AIFS.

Helitzer, D. L., Cunningham-Sabo, L. D., Van Leit, B., & Crowe, T. K. (2002). Perceived changes in self-image and coping strategies of mothers of children with disabilities. *Occupational Therapy Journal of Research, 22*, 25–33.

Koltyn, K. F., & Schultes, S. S. (1997). Psychological effects of an aerobic exercise session and a rest session following pregnancy. *Journal of Sports Medicine and Physical Fitness, 37*, 287–291.

Lenz, E. R., Parks, P. L., Jenkins, L. S., & Jarrett, G. E. (1986). Life change and instrumental support as predictors of illness in mothers of 6-month olds. *Research in Nursing & Health, 9*, 17–24.

Littlewood, J., & McHugh, N. (1997). *Maternal distress and postnatal depression. The myth of madonna*. Basingstoke, UK: Macmillan.

Maushart, S. (1997). *The mask of motherhood. How motherhood changes everything and why we pretend it doesn't*. Milson's Point, Sydney: Random House.

Mercer, R. (1995). *Becoming a mother. Research on maternal identity from Rubin to the present*. New York: Springer.

Michelson, W. (1985). *From sun to sun: Daily obligations and community structure in the lives of employed women and their families*. New Jersey, US: Rowman & Allanheld.

Milkie, M. A., Bianchi, S. M., Mattingly, M. J., & Robinson, J. P. (2002). Gendered division of childrearing: Ideals, realities, and the relationship to parental well-being. *Sex Roles, 47*, 21–38.

Mullin, E., Quigley, K., & Glanville, B. (1994). A controlled evaluation of the impact of a parent-training program on child behavior and mother's general well-being. *Counselling Psychology Quarterly, 7,* 167–179.

Mulsow, M., Caldera, Y. M., Pursley, M., Reifman, A., & Huston, A. C. (2002). Multilevel factors influencing maternal stress during the first three years. *Journal of Marriage & the Family, 64,* 944–956.

Musil, C. M., & Abraham, I. L. (1986). Coping, thinking, and mental health nursing: Cognitions and their application to psychosocial intervention. *Issues in Mental Health Nursing, 8,* 191–210.

Oakley, A. (1979). *Becoming A mother*. Oxford: Robinson.

O'Hara, M. W., Schlechte, J. A., Lewis, D. A., & Varner, M. W. (1995). Controlled prospective study of postpartum mood disorders: Psychological, environmental, and hormonal variables. *Journal of Abnormal Psychology, 100,* 63–73.

Phoenix, A, Woollett, A, & Lloyd, E. (1991). *Motherhood. meanings, practices and ideology.* London: Sage.

Prokos, A. H. (2003). A new kind of father? Progressive fathers and gender differentiation. *Southern Sociological Society (USA) Association Paper*, 2003S41165.

Raskin, P. M., Kummel, P., & Bannister, T. (1998). The relationship between coping styles, attachment, and career salience in partnered working women with children. *Journal of Career Assessment, 6,* 403–416.

Sampselle, C., Seng, J., Yeo, S., Killion, C., & Oakley, D. (1999). Physical activity and postpartum well-being. *Journal of Obstetric, Gynecological and neonatal Nursing, 28,* 41–49.

Scott, M., & Stradling, S. G. (1987). Evaluation of a group program for parents of problem children. *Behavioral Psychotherapy, 15,* 224–239.

Sethi, S. (1995). The dialectic in becoming a mother: Experiencing a postpartum phenomenon. *Scandinavian Journal of Caring Science, 9,* 235–244.

Todres, R., & Bunston, T. (1993). Parent-education program evaluation: A review of the literature. *Canadian Journal of Mental Health, 12,* 225–257.

Tudor, K. (1999). *Mental health promotion*. London: Routledge.

Tulman, L., Fawcett, J., Groblewski, L., & Silverman, L. (1990). Changes in functional status after childbirth. *Nursing Research, 39,* 70–75.

Walker, L., & Wilging, S. (2000). Rediscovering the "M" in "MCH": Maternal health promotion after childbirth. *Journal of Obstetric, Gynaecologic and Neonatal Nursing, 29,* 229–236.

Wearing, B. (1984). *The ideology of motherhood*. Sydney: George Allen and Unwin.

Wearing, B. (1990). Leisure and the crisis of motherhood: A study of leisure and health amongst mothers of first babies in Sydney, Australia. In S. R. Quah (Ed.), *The family as an asset: An international perspective on marriage* (pp. 122–155). Singapore: Times Academic Press.

Welles-Nystrom, B., New, R., & Richman, A. (1994). The 'good mother': a comparative study of Swedish, Italian and American maternal behavior and goals. *Scandinavian Journal of Caring Sciences, 8,* 81–86.

Chapter 4
The Meaning and Lived Experience of Coping

> *Coping is just being able to keep going day-to-day and keep looking after them without falling to pieces, which sometimes can be really difficult. I was just really, really tired, and you just have to keep going because they don't stop, so you just keep going.* (Wendy)

Abstract According to the mothers, coping equates with feeling a sense of control. Feeling in control is like being on auto-pilot and getting things done. Mothers can cope to different degrees or levels. However, mothers are more aware of the times when they feel they're coping at lower levels. The main aspects of their everyday life they cope with on a daily basis include the pressure of having to appear as coping, the drastic change in lifestyle after having a baby, and that the fact mothering is simply a difficult role with lots of challenges and obligations.

4.1 Introduction

This chapter categorises the meaning of coping in everyday living, as explained by the group of mothers I interviewed for this book. According to the mothers, coping includes a feeling of control of one's situation. This is consistent with the theoretical context of this study that health promotion includes increasing people's control over their own health and lifestyle (Currie, 2008).

This chapter also presents the day-to-day situations nominated by the mothers as the events and challenges they feel they need to cope with. The mothers described a complex array of experiences and pressures they cope with. The rich descriptions provided to illustrate the categories identified reinforce the value of qualitatively investigating the meaning of coping.

© The Author(s) 2018
J. L. Currie, *Managing Motherhood*, SpringerBriefs in Well-Being and Quality of Life Research, https://doi.org/10.1007/978-981-13-0338-8_4

4.2   Insights to the Lived Experience of Coping

When attempting to define what coping means to mothers of young children, the qualitative findings revealed two main themes. Coping or effectively managing motherhood involves:

- Feeling in control, and
- Degrees of coping: higher and lower levels of coping.

4.2.1   Feeling in Control

The first theme to emerge which helped to define what coping meant from the mothers' own point of view, was related to a feeling in control of one's situation. Bruess and Richardson (1989) also described effective coping as being in control or managing external events. Trish described this scenario as when she feels she's operating on auto-pilot; "It's wonderful! Feels like everything is cruising along". On the other hand, Sarah felt that in general, mothers could never achieve a state of 'total' control when attempting to cope:

> No, I don't think you ever have control when you have children because it changes from minute to minute and they really control your day. So there's never total control, I think.

Congruent with a feeling of being on auto-pilot, mothers tended to be less aware or to not even notice during the times they were coping:

> …you don't even think about it at all. You don't, like, you don't often get up and think, 'Well, I'm coping today', unless something happens, the feeling that you're not, rather than you are. (Trish)

Coping or feeling in control was also commonly related by the mothers to a feeling of 'getting things done', as explained by Trish, Sarah and Kate:

> Just a bit of everything; having everything run smoothly, being reasonably happy and all the important things around the house are done and are looked after, really. I'm a very organised person and that's how I like it to be, and I guess if I wasn't organising things and getting them done, then I guess I'd feel like I wasn't coping. (Trish)

> The house would be in some kind of order. We could find our clothes, and um, meals are on the table at a time that I can then get the kids into a bath and into bed, and those things run smoothly, those day to day things… If I have some sort of routine happening, where I have 2–3 days at home…where she gets a good sleep in and I get my boring housework and my washing and ironing done, then I feel like I cope. If I have a week where I go out and blow that routine out the window, then I don't feel like I cope at all, and then I get stressed and then I start yelling at them and expecting things of them they're not capable of. If I try to do more than the everyday stuff with them, I don't cope, whereas if I go one day at a time with them, I cope. (Sarah)

> I think coping has to include getting things done, because that's really what you've got to do; have your house clean, your children happy. (Kate)

In contrast, the mothers in this study were more aware of the intense feelings they experienced when *not* coping, as explained by Vanessa:

> It's a contrast really, when you're coping you're on auto-pilot, but when you're having a bad day, you've got more stress, and I might get to the end of the day and think, 'Oh no, I shouted at him too much today', and feel really bad and that sort of thing. On the good days or normal days, I don't get to the end of the day and think, 'Oh wow, that was a really good day', or if I feel something really special has happened, then I might feel that was a really good day. But generally, day-to-day, I don't really think, 'Oh, I've got through the day', or anything like that, I just go ahead and do it, I don't dwell on it too much. (Vanessa)

Cynthia could detect feelings of 'not coping' when her nerves were fraying and her patience was running out:

> I often think of it, actually. I know when I'm coping badly, and that's usually when I can see my patience running out and I'm short tempered – that's when I know I'm not coping. (Cynthia)

Phillipa found it easier to be consciously aware of times when she wasn't coping due to the distinctly negative contrast:

> I don't notice when I'm coping, I only notice when I'm not coping because I'm sort of on edge. That's when things feel out of control, and when I'm down and I get angry and might lose it with the kids, as opposed to being able to sort of manage it. (Phillipa)

Coping also involved the mother providing opportunities for quality time together with her family and contributing to their personal development:

> Just get on with it, really. Um, I guess Mitchell's my priority, so he has to come first, and to make sure my husband's kept happy, that there's food on the table and prepared, and the cleaning and all of those sorts of things are done. But also that I have some quality time with him and that he gets the best opportunity to learn and develop, and I suppose remember that he's only two and a half and not get sort of too strung out when he's having a bad day. (Vanessa)

That is, according to the mothers, in addition to completing all of the usual household tasks, coping meant that everybody around them was feeling happy and receiving all the attention and nurturing they needed. The mothers coped by completing chores and having time left for nurturing others, as explained by these two mothers:

> It's just a matter of doing it [household chores] and making sure that everyone around you is happy and your child's getting what she needs and um, and I suppose your husband's getting what he needs and you're not getting stressed out, and it's just a matter of doing it. (Kate)

> I feel on top of things, if the house is kind of clean and I don't have mounds of washing or anything around me. And if my kids are happy, if Robert sounds like he's not being hardly done by, he's having a friend over occasionally, you know, getting to the park a bit, that sort of stuff, if those things run smoothly, things can pretty much fall into place. (Sarah)

However, when attempting to 'get everything done', mothers desired to also experience the positive element of quality or balance. The following response from Cynthia highlighted the importance of experiencing some love and fun, and not constantly finding day-to-day events to be pure drudgery:

> I tend to think of coping as functioning reasonably well, getting things done, um, but we're still talking basics, aren't we? Loving them is an important thing, you don't want it just to be a drudgery, to look at it like that, because this is such an important time in their life as well, and you want to input love and fun, and those sorts of things as well. (Cynthia)

When attempting to complete daily tasks, meet everyone's needs and still achieve a balance, Cynthia mentioned the importance of finding some time-out for self:

> Yeah, I think coping is that you're feeling that you're getting a balance of everything, you're getting enough of the so called jobs done, everyone's happy, and that's really important; everyone, their needs are being met, and that you do also have some free time as well. Often that's the one thing that you just don't get to do.

So being an effective time-manager is important because it helps the mother have some remaining time for herself after all of the other tasks are complete.

4.2.2   Different Levels or Degrees of Coping

The second theme to emerge was the ability of the mothers to experience different levels of coping. Lower levels were still regarded as coping per se. However, it was not considered as efficacious, or as effective or empowering an experience as high-level, 'cruise-control' coping. Wendy explained this concept:

> Yeah, I think there's different levels of coping. Like you can survive, and just get by, or you can feel really on top of things and really confident in what you're doing, and I would say when we were going through their waking we were just surviving, um, but it was stressful, and neither of us felt good, and, but now that it's more under control...Just hanging on, you feel dreadful, stressed, powerless in a lot of ways, um where, kind of where I am now, which is kind of more than just surviving, um, I feel a lot more confident in what I'm doing and in being able to approach what they're doing. I think a lot of it has to do with confidence and feeling assured of what's going on. (Wendy)

A mother can cope, but she may describe this as just 'scraping through' at a low level of coping or basic survival level. 'Higher' levels of coping were described as achieving the most satisfaction, enjoyment and happiness:

> Coping to me is just getting by, I guess, up to feeling happy and fulfilled and accomplishing what I want to accomplish. (Kate)

> I think when I'm coping, I think of the enjoyment level. Thinking, 'This is good, this is OK, I love my children'. (Cynthia)

According to Phillipa, a vital ingredient of being able to cope at higher levels included finding some time-out for yourself:

> Getting through the day, getting everything done that needs to be done for the family and the house and yourself, that's just coping. Beyond coping is where you can do something for yourself as well, I think. A higher level of coping.

The next section describes some of the situations that the mothers coped with in their day-to-day lifestyle.

4.3 What Do Mothers Say They Cope with?

When attempting to explain the situations mothers felt they needed to cope with on a day-to-day basis, three main themes emerged from the qualitative data, including:

- Pressure to appear as coping; an ideal mother image
- Lifestyle changes experienced since the baby was born
- The difficulty of the mothering role.

The themes related to key ideas around the mothers' philosophy of mothering. There appeared to be a strong perception among these women that social pressure was high and they willingly/unwillingly strived to fit the ideal, or justify why they couldn't.

4.3.1 Experiencing Pressures to 'Have to Appear as Coping'

The mothers in this study were aware of an image or ideology of having to appear as though they were coping at all times. Henderson, Bialeschki, Shaw, and Freysinger (1989, pp. 24–25) explained how social indoctrination imposed on women a value system stating that if they are to be a 'good' mother, they must put their family first. Further, the role of wife and mother is the highest expression and recognition of their femininity. Typical responses describing these perceived social pressures and ideal images included:

> I definitely think there's an image of what a mother should be. A mother should cope, that they should be able to perk themselves up no matter what they're facing. (Wendy)

> Yeah, I think it's a personal thing, but for me, I like to have a tidy house, even if I only see it, I feel conscious of it. Everybody round you expects your children to be quiet and well behaved and you to be coping and they expect you to accomplish that no matter whether you're having a good day or a bad day. You have to cope with how your parents feel, you know, how you should be bringing up children; coping with everybody's ideas about how children should behave. (Kate)

> …but I think [I have to cope with] just external pressures to perform. You know, to be seen as being together, I don't know. There's a lot of pressure on you. I do feel outside pressures, they're probably just me thinking they're coming from the outside, but it's with the housework and the way the house is, you know, I never thought was important and I know theoretically it isn't. It's just amazing how that can play a role in your expectations. I've developed them, I was never conscious of it, it's such a superficial concern and still, but I think there is such a pervasive mentality or expectation of appearance which is on everything, the body, your kids, how well dressed your children are, it's all around here. (Cynthia)

At the end of the day, Vanessa explained to me how she believed that it was individually up to her to find ways to cope:

> I suppose you sort of expect that you have to put up with a certain amount of stress. During the day you just think that's what being a mother's all about. I still think the mother gets most of the coping, you know, Mark's quite good with Mitchell and things like that, but at the end of the day, it's up to me to deal with everything.

According to Wendy, to have to ask for help was tantamount to not coping or admitting defeat:

> Because of the image, if you ask for help, you're not coping, and you're not good enough. But it's so strong, and so many people won't say, I left one mothers' group because they all seemed to have perfect babies and none of them were happy to talk about what was hard and what was difficult or what you got sick of. Their babies couldn't be as perfect or as plastic as they were making out they were. (Wendy)

4.3.2 Life's 'Different' Now

All mothers mentioned a drastic lifestyle change that needed to be adjusted to since the birth of the baby. This was consistently described as quite a 'shock'. These two mothers help to explain this phenomenon:

> It's really different! [laughs] I think after 5 years, I'm just getting used to it. A drastic change. I have spats when I try to remember what it was like back then because I want to remember what it felt like to be normal. I don't think I am any more (laughs). (Sarah)

> Well I think it [becoming a mum] was a great shock, but it was a great thrill. I was delighted of course, but I don't think I've had such great challenges in my life since being a mum. (Cynthia)

In becoming mothers, women experience a major transition involving contradictions, tensions and transformations. Although happy to become mothers, at the same time women lose significant freedom, autonomy, and predictability (Sethi, 1995, p. 235).

Similarly, all of the mothers I interviewed for this book described contrasting lifestyles experienced pre- to post-baby, such as less time to self, loss of freedom and dealing with a difficult toddler. Cynthia described the change for her in terms of a change in self-identity:

> I just think the great shock of… you lose identity, you're no longer you know, a such and such, you're no longer this and that, you're suddenly a mother, there's a real identity change.

Life was different, because the mothers now spent their time caring for others:

> It's busy, busy, um, it's hard to describe because you're so focused on what you're doing that it's hard… that what I did before, I was busy then, but now it's just different, that everything is to do with them, and any time I have away from them has to do with them. So yeah, like I used to work full-time and be out most nights, so now I've got a couple of little things I do during the week but the rest of the time is spent at home. So there's not as much contact with people outside, um, yeah, it's just busy. And like on weekends, there's no holiday, there's no break, yeah, so that's different to what it was. As I said, I'm not going out as much, whereas before home was somewhere we just visited to sleep (laughs). (Wendy)

> I guess I'm a stay-at-home mum now. I was working full-time before as a computer programmer and it's quite a lifestyle change. Um, Mitchell keeps me pretty busy… It's not easy work, but it's different, 20 h a day as opposed to 9 to 5 or whatever. It's different kinds of stressors. Obviously in the workplace you're dealing with clients and colleagues and things like that, meeting deadlines and corporate type stuff, whereas dealing with a toddler, it's a

different mentality. You're dealing with tantrums, you know, keeping him busy, 'What do I do now?' Especially days like today when it's pouring. Some days you just go stir crazy. (Vanessa)

Sarah explained this concept as not "even having a life anymore":

Bloody hell, yeah [life's different]. I don't have a life anymore. It's just completely different, you live and breathe for them, and there isn't much room for anything else. (Sarah)

All mothers agreed that motherhood did result in a perceived loss of personal freedom.

I've had to cope with loss of freedom, for example. We used to sail our boat competitively and do a lot of racing and stuff like that; I guess it hit home during the pregnancy…. (Trish)

At the focus group with all mothers present, Kate said how she thought that the hardest change to deal with after having children was the lack of time for self:

Oh yeah [life before children], it's just an ideal, isn't it? (laughs) Just to be able to sort of say to yourself, 'I'm so tired, I'm going to have half an hour time-out'. Now you don't get that any more. And I think that's the hardest thing to deal with, that lack of self-time.

4.3.3   Difficulty of Mothering

The shock of becoming a mother also entailed adaptation to how difficult the role is, as explained by these three informants:

Yeah, you're gonna find that it's all a bit much to start with, and you're a nappy changing, feeding machine, and you're doing something for one, and then the other, then your husband comes home or whatever. I'm sure you're gonna feel a little more stressed and like you're not coping as well. (Trish)

Certainly the first thing you have to cope with is the babies and what they dish out, whether it be sickness, whether it be difficult sleeping patterns, whether it be just a whole range of things. That's the first thing you have to cope with, um, then trying to balance that with any other external demands, so whether it be, friends, family, work, that will be later, so yeah, and dealing with everything that comes outside. (Wendy)

I cope with trying to get everything done by the end of the day, especially with two children, and trying to give them some attention through the day, and also getting everything else done. Yeah, pretty well my life revolves around Mitchell, and Adam just fits in at the moment. (Vanessa)

The informants stated how everyday they generally, on a day-to-day basis, had to cope with demands arising from all fronts:

I have to cope with everything. I think you really have to cope with the demands of your children and the demands of your partner, cope with the demands of the outside world, and the demands of your children. (Kate)

Cynthia often coped on her own for 6 weeks at a time while her husband was away at work. She also felt like she had to balance her outside commitments with home demands:

I think primarily, because Stephen goes away it's different, because he goes away for 6 weeks, I really am doing the finances, and I find that a bit of a burden. Running around, it doesn't sound like much, but just trying to keep the house tidy, the bills paid, just functioning on a basic level. And then trying to maintain relationships outside of family, I guess that's what's led to the voluntary work. I find that's a dilemma, am I using my energy up on others outside the family and are my immediate family being short-changed?

Sarah described juggling the demands of new motherhood as being a difficult, baby-focused task. There is so much work to do in the time available:

Sometimes, although I'm home all day, sometimes at the end of the day, I think, 'There's not enough hours in the day', so I feel like I'm coping with trying to fit in all the things I want to do...and Michelle was only six or eight months or something, and she was on my hip the whole time I was doing work...that was really, really hard, and I found that I was constantly torn between what I should and shouldn't be doing, and not doing it well. That's what it comes down to, I think, trying to do too much with a baby, and you don't do anything well. I think it's really hard being a mum. And because you're being tested all the time by them, and I don't think I have that patience and that natural maternity thing where you desperately want to do that, so I guess I find it a trying experience, good, obviously, but trying.

During the early period of motherhood, women often experience common problems such as loss of sleep, tiredness, increased household chores, and loss of freedom (Martin, 1995). The demands of juggling tasks meant that the mother felt her own needs being squeezed or neglected, as explained by Kate:

Oh yeah, it gets a bit much, when you spend your whole life trying to get things done for the baby, what they need, and getting things done for the children. I've got 3 children, so I'm very baby-focused, and there's not much room for you and your partner. (Kate)

Phillipa explained that there was a multitude of tasks to complete on a daily basis. However, she noted that if she coped, the end result was invisible, or not necessarily noticed by others. She felt that the results of coping were less visible than evidence of not coping:

Coping with keeping a family in order. Coping with making sure there's bread and milk and all those things that need to be at home and making sure the washing's kept up to date and then the other bits and pieces of keeping a household like paying bills and making phone calls to whoever and all those household affairs, and it's amazing how many things you have to do with each day, and how my husband will come home and say, 'What did you do today?', and um, I give up sort of itemising things, now I say, 'Nothing interesting', or 'Nothing out of the ordinary', even though I know I didn't sit down once and relax. It's like a blur, it's not visible, is it? There's much more evidence of not coping or not dealing with things as opposed to feeling as though you're coping.

The mother's role in nurturing and keeping everyone in the household happy was a consistently reported issue that informants had to confront daily:

I think you do feel that you're the one that has to keep everyone happy, and in doing so you don't think about your own needs. You do put everyone first, and make sure they're happy. (Trish)

You know that the relationship with your husband has got to function [in addition to that with the children]. The health of your relationship with your spouse will affect the relationship with your children. If you're tense, fighting and unhappy, that'll affect your children. I've heard that it's the woman who dictates the atmosphere of the home. (Cynthia)

4.4 Conclusion

According to the mothers, coping equated with a sense of 'feeling in control' of one's situation. Coping was able to be experienced at high and low levels. Low-level coping included a feeling of just getting by, while high-level coping involved a sense of quality, enjoyment and hopefully some time-out for self. While coping with everyday mothering tasks was perceived as challenging and even difficult at times, an element of quality was deemed important. Therefore it was considered important that daily lifestyles should not become a life of total drudgery. As Cynthia said, "getting a balance" or "having some free time as well" was as important as "getting things done".

The mothers were more aware of the feelings experienced when not coping compared with times when they were coping. That is, the mothers described how they weren't as consciously aware of when they *were* coping. "I don't notice when I'm coping, I only notice when I'm not coping because I'm sort of on edge" (Phillipa). The mothers could distinctly detect the contrast between a sense of coping and not coping, mainly due to the stressful feeling of not coping. As Vanessa said, "when you're coping you're on auto-pilot, but when you have a bad day, you've got more stress" (Vanessa). Not coping was described as "patience running out...short tempered" (Cynthia). This contrasts with Trish's description for coping as "managing the situation, getting things done".

Perhaps adding to the mothers' stress levels, when taking on the burden of running a household, the mothers felt great responsibility for the emotional health of all those around them. For example, Cynthia mentioned how "I've heard that it is the woman who dictates the atmosphere of the home" (Cynthia). While at the focus group, Kate said she felt responsible for "making sure that everyone around you is happy".

The mothers were aware of social pressures to conform to an ideal image and appear as coping effectively at all times. "Because of the image, if you ask for help, you're not coping, and you're not good enough" (Wendy). Typically, perception of a social pressure to perform well or cope as a mother was also described as "extreme pressure to perform" (Cynthia). Kate said "I feel conscious of it... everybody round you expects you to be coping" while Wendy asserted "I definitely think there's an image of what a mother should be".

The mothers had experienced a major "shock" caused by drastic lifestyle changes experienced since the birth of their babies and had to adapt to a new role. Sarah concluded; "I try to remember what it was like back then [before the baby] because I want to remember what it felt like to be normal". Mothers felt like they were on 24 h stand-by with little time to self. The mothers expressed a feeling of coping with multiple demands. Time was spent focusing on others, and the mothering role was often described as busy, challenging and difficult. It may be in teaching other household members to be more self-sufficient, or in expanding the role of fathers or partners to include more caring, that the mothers may feel a break from this feeling of being on-call.

New motherhood is a difficult period of adjustment for women. "I don't think I've had such great challenges in my life since being a mum" (Cynthia). "Some days you just go stir crazy" (Vanessa). The post-baby challenges were immense but the mothers were stoic and resilient in their adaptation and coping.

Perhaps all they needed was more time-out to themselves, because "…you spend your whole life trying to get things done for the baby…there's not much room for you and your partner" (Kate). Trish mentioned how she had to mainly cope now with "the loss of freedom", and Kate said that for her, "that's the hardest thing to deal with, that lack of freedom".

Despite the pressures, there appeared to be little social recognition of the mothers' coping efforts. The findings contained in this chapter also revealed a current of dissatisfaction or wanting by the mothers to be recognised for a job well done. For example, Phillipa concluding that coping's "not visible", and "there's much more evidence of not-coping".

Coping was important to the mothers. It was related to having confidence in one's role. For example, Wendy said when she was coping, "I feel a lot more confident in what I'm doing and in being able to approach what they're doing". This contrasted with her perceptions of less effective coping, such as "…you feel dreadful, stressed, powerless in a lot of ways" (Wendy). All mothers had developed coping strategies in an attempt to deal with perceived stressors. These strategies are reviewed in Chap. 5.

References

Bruess, C., & Richardson, G. (1989). *Decisions for health* (2nd ed.). Dubuque, IA: WM C. Brown.
Currie, J. L. (2008). Conditions affecting perceived coping for new mothers: Analysis of a pilot study, Sydney, Australia. *The International Journal of Mental Health Promotion, 10,* 34–41.
Henderson, K. A., Bialeschki, M. D., Shaw, S. M., & Freysinger, V. J. (1989). *A leisure of one's own: A feminist perspective on women's leisure.* PA, US: Venture.
Martin, B. P. (1995). *An analysis of common postpartum problems and adaptation strategies used by women during the first two to eight weeks following delivery of a fullterm, healthy newborn.* Unpublished Ph.D. thesis, University of Mississippi.
Sethi, S. (1995). The dialectic in becoming a mother: Experiencing a postpartum phenomenon. *Scandinavian Journal of Caring Science, 9,* 235–244.

Chapter 5
Strategies Used to Manage Motherhood

It's just willing to be open, to say when you're not coping, 'Can you please help me?'. I think it's a difficult thing to do, of course I'll tell my mum I need help, but I think that it's hard to ask other people outside (Cynthia).

Abstract The main strategies mothers say they use to cope with their role include obtaining outside help, having a plan or routine, and escaping with time-out. At the end of the day, if a mother doesn't take control and cope, there was no-one else to step in. Who nurtures and cares for mothers? Asking for help could be construed as not coping. If taking in help or being nurtured leads to greater well-being, mothers may need to be more open and willing to seeking out and accessing resources, help and assistance more often.

5.1 Introduction

The purpose of this book is to illustrate in detail the strategies mothers of young children say they use to cope with their everyday lifestyle. This chapter details the coping strategies identified by the mothers I interviewed as the ones that helped them deal with their day-to-day lifestyles. The qualitative data helps to contextualise the coping experience and provide insight into details of the preferred ways of coping. The three main themes to arise from the qualitative data illustrating how mothers cope with their role included:

- Obtaining outside help
- Having a plan or schedule which helped establish routine and organisation
- Time-out or escape from normal duties.

5.2   Obtaining Outside Help

All of the mothers I interviewed mentioned to me that seeking or obtaining help from others was a method that currently assisted them or would potentially assist them to cope. According to Kahn (1979) and Tarkka, Paunonen, and Laippala (1996), social support can take the form of affect (appreciation, admiration, love), affirmation (reinforcement, feedback, information influencing decisions), and concrete (providing objects, money, help and time). Dunkel-Schetter, Blasband, Feinstein, and Bennett (1992) described emotional support (acceptance and understanding), informational support (advice and problem-solving) and instrumental assistance (aiding with tasks or contributing materials) as the three main categories of social support or help. In Bennett's (1981) survey, new mothers sought childcare advice, occasional help with baby-sitting, and instrumental or practical help, such as hiring a cleaner.

My informants explained to me how husbands or partners and the mother's own mother were potential sources of support. The following four informants' descriptions typified this category:

> A lot of people seem to have a lot of help, or their husbands home early in the afternoons, and that's how they cope, because they've got that extra assistance, and I reckon if you could have that, life would be a hell of a lot easier. (Sarah)

> Having Bill as support certainly makes things a lot easier than they would be otherwise, and knowing where I can turn to have somebody to talk to and come up with ideas, that's really helpful as well. (Wendy)

> Oh yeah, just being able to have a shower or just the very simple things, knowing that he's in there supervising them while I get dinner! Even as a friend was saying today, she'd know the time she was starting to lose her temper and she could just say to her husband, 'Take them away', and she said, 'How do you cope with that?' [not having your husband always available] and I said 'not very well, a lot of the time, and I can tell when I'm starting to really lose it'. Family support's important, having a break at some stage during the day, and when Stephen's away, Mum will come for a morning or whatever, and I will go out, and yeah, I think that's essential. I think it's refreshing and you just come back and are glad to see the children again, whereas before, it's like, 'Get them away!'. (Cynthia)

> My mum arrives on Saturday and that'll be a great help. She's very efficient around the house. She's good with *children* too, so she'll be a great help. She's staying for 8 weeks. (Vanessa)

Where available, mothers seemed to be able to freely ask their own mothers for help without feeling too much guilt as a consequence:

> Yeah, I don't have my mum close by and it is much easier to ask your own mum. (Trish)

> My mum, initially I didn't think she'd come down during school holidays, she comes after work, she's a teacher, but she loves it so much, that she loves being with them so much, she comes anyway. So that for her, I know it's not an imposition, it's not a huge deal for her. (Wendy)

Sarah indicated that she would like to ask her mother to help, but was unable to as she lived too far away:

> I would be able to ask my mum or mother-in-law [for help], because I know that they'd enjoy it as well, but I'd feel a bit guilty asking my sister because she's got kids of her own to worry

about. I think having a bit of help is what other women do. And I think that's where I get stressed because I don't have any back-up at all. (Sarah)

All informants with mothers located geographically distant did not have access to this source of outside help. Compared with her friends, Sarah stated how she felt hard done by in that she perceived her support network to be less than that of her peers. She did not have the back-up of her mother. She related to me at other times during her interview, how her husband did not support her adequately either. He was described more in terms of being the breadwinner of the family. Sarah may have felt vulnerable and wanted to be parented herself. Parents who feel a close bond or attachment with their own parents usually report greater levels of social support during parenting from their own parents and others (Feeney, 2002). The lack of social capital and support networks more prevalent in today's society may be due to the loss of extended families, divorce, and geographical or other barriers such as a grandmother's perception of preferring a reduced role. It may mean that some mothers miss out more on the nurturing one can receive from one's own parent/s, especially the mother's own mother.

Other sources of help included talking with an understanding friend or even a healthcare professional:

I think finding the external support [helps me cope]. Being able to, when you're in a difficult situation, of finding somebody to talk to that can offer suggestions or just act as a sounding board; that's been really important to me, that at 2 o'clock in the morning, I've been able to phone one of the support lines and say, 'Right, let's go through this, this is what I've tried. These are all the different things, where do I go to, what else can I try?'. (Wendy)

Vanessa highlighted her perception of the need for support by peers:

I think having other people around with children of similar ages is really a help, like Mothers Group or Playgroup, or the Pramwalkers. Just because, it's nice to have adult company at some stage during the day and you can share experiences and concerns and things like that. You find out you're not the only one with a certain kind of issue, whatever, everybody's going through the same thing. And also the children enjoy each other's company, especially at this age, they enjoy each other's company a lot more and they seem to be a lot happier when they've got each other around. (Vanessa)

Wendy and Cynthia had similar stories:

I go walking with a girl who's got twins, but they're two weeks younger. We were living in the unit block next door to each other, and were pregnant, and so we talk a lot about what's going on and gain support. And so that's good. She's got no family support, whereas I've got lots. Just to have somebody who understands the demands of having two babies and that when you get one to sleep, that's only half the story. (Wendy)

I think through talking to other mothers, you have more of an idea on how to deal with certain issues. That helps. (Cynthia)

Sometimes, even though asking for help may seem like the best thing to do, the mother may not be able to bring herself to actually ask for or admit she needs help. For this group of mothers, asking for help induced feelings of awkwardness, obligation or guilt, as explained by the following three mothers:

...I think you need to be able to see someone to talk and ask for help. Predominantly for me, it's from people I have to be ready to ask. I know I should avail myself of people more from my church. You know, when Stephen's away, just say, 'Please, come and help me!' People have offered, well the lady up the road, but it's hard, you feel like you're imposing on them. I think information, of course is so valuable, and I think it's often difficult, because I think everyone's experience differs, really, but I think talking, really, and just communicating with other mums, with grandmothers, with whomever. I just found a community health nurse down at Ashby – fabulous! That's a fabulous facility we have. It's just willing to be open, to say when you're not coping, 'Can you please help me? I think it's a difficult thing to do, of course I'll tell my mum I need help, but I think that it's hard to ask other people outside. (Cynthia)

But I think one of the more personal things is being able to ask for help. And that, I would say, is a problem that I have, is that I don't ask. I'd be comfortable to ask my mum, husband or dad or sister, but outside of that, even when it's offered, I find it hard to accept it. (Phillipa)

You've got to have someone to ask, if you don't have a mum, there's no one else you feel comfortable about asking. If you ask friends, you've got to help them back in return, and it never seems to be at a convenient time, but that's just something you've got to wear because they've done the right thing by you. It's just awkward; I don't like to ask people for help. (Sarah)

The strength of a mother's social ties, network and support may assist her to seek out help, be it of a health information nature, or practical help around the home (Carpentier & White, 2002; Reifman & Dunkel-Schetter, 1990). Prevalent reasons for women not seeking out medical help in a study by Peters and Bayer (1999) were the existence of a waiting list, lack of motivation or resolution of the health problem. Therefore, this suggests that the informants may not be 'desperate' enough yet to have to ask for help to cope with housework, for example, or they may believe they have any problems under control.

However, not asking for help could be related to mothers not personally identifying as failing or being 'sick'. The General Practitioners commenting on patients in a study by De Nooijer, Lechner, and De Vries (2001) mentioned lack of knowledge and fear as barriers to help-seeking behaviours. Their findings vindicate the mothers in this book who felt unable to ask for help as it would label them as not coping or failing in their role on their own, to others, themselves, or both.

For the research informants, if one had the means, paying for help was definitely viewed as an attractive option:

If I could afford to pay for help I would have someone come in once or twice a week and I could go out and do my walks. For me, even once a week for a couple of hours would be good, just a little bit of help. (Sarah)

However, at the focus group interview, Kate stated that although it would be her "dream" to be able to access paid help, the thought of going to work to earn the extra money necessary to pay for it was not an attractive option:

If we had a lot of spare money, we'd get outside help for sure for the family's well-being as much as to the mother's well-being. But then the only way to get that is to go out and work and then as soon as you work, it eats into your time. For me it's a dream thing. (Kate)

Previous studies also point to financial stress creating barriers to accessing leisure or time-out options (Rhodes, 1982), while a positive relationship exists between recreation expenditures and income (Dardis, Derrick, Lehfeld, & Wolfe, 1981). Further, women who "only work in the home have no personal income, little power or prestige, and low status in society" (Henderson et al., 1989, p. 121).

At the focus group, Ann thought that outside help or support was particularly important for the new mother with a very young baby. She described new mothers as being on their 'L Plates' [Learner's Driver's Licence], or being at the early stages of a learning experience. She said the new mother may feel more like she is on her 'L plates' and may either not know how to deal with situations as they arise or know what is normal:

> I think having back-up is very important to a new mother. I didn't have a lot of back-up as far as family [when I had my baby], but I had a close friend who would ring nearly every day and pop in as much as possible. But um, it's really hard because you don't know what to expect and you're on your L plates and you don't know how to deal with it, um, it would be good if you had a clinic sister just to come in, just to tell you or some sort of back-up system, whether it's Play Group, Mother's Group or whatever, just to let you know that what you're going through at the time is normal and don't have too many high expectations.

The ideas raised by Ann support the notion of access to 'Parenting Education', highly reported in the literature for its successful outcomes with supporting teenage mothers. Fang and Frizzell (1998) found that after participating in a parenting education program, both parents showed an increase in several areas of adjustment. Mothers reported a statistically significant decrease in parenting stress related to feeling restricted or loss of freedom, and a perceived increase in social support, whereas fathers reported statistically significant increases in marital adjustment and a reduction of parenting stress related to competence.

Other benefits of meeting other mothers at Mothers' Groups can include increased sense of social support. Wendy recommended against other mothers "going it alone" or not asking for help when it was ideally required:

> I wouldn't recommend going it alone. Relying on just you, like not talking to your partner, trying to be the stalwart. It just doesn't work.

A study of 150 mothers of infants and toddlers with disabilities found that participants in professionally organised parent groups reported larger increases in the size and helpfulness of their social support networks than did non-participants (Krauss & Wyngaarden, 1993).

5.3   Having a Plan or Schedule

Having a plan or being organised was recommended by this group of mothers as helping them coping more effectively with daily tasks, as illustrated by these three responses:

> I guess I'm reasonably organised, like I have a bit of a routine in the morning and get up and have a shower, make the lunches for Dave, do breakfast, put the washing on, and get that out of the way. And then we'll do something in the morning and go out hopefully, and he

doesn't have any sleep in the afternoons any more, but at least have some quiet time in the afternoon, and that's when I'll catch up on some housework. So fairly routined, and that's my strategy of coping, just having a routine, not a rigid one that works by the clock, unless I have an appointment or something like that, but there's an evident routine. (Vanessa)

I find routine is how I cope. Routine. It works well if you're out the door at the same time everyday, if you have her having a sleep at the same time every day. Those sorts of things. It makes them fit into your structure and therefore you tend to cope a lot better. That's what I find works. (Sarah)

For me it's mainly being organised, that's my way of coping. If I feel I've got up and made the beds or washed up or something, you know, set things in their place and the place is reasonably tidy and then it's my little way of coping. (Trish)

Routines often helped mothers cope as they felt more efficient in their whole approach, got more chores completed so had fewer tasks 'hanging over' them or left to do. Making an early start to the day was one way mothers said helped them to cope or feel 'on top of things':

...as far as day to day things go, I try to get organised at the beginning of the day, you know, I like to get things done. I don't like things hanging over me. So we'll try and get breakfast and washing out of the way first thing in the morning, and try and get out and have a play with Mitchell in the mornings, then get the chores done in the afternoon, get the dinner. So things are fairly structured in that way. (Vanessa)

I'm a creature of habit, and routine, and I like to feel on top of things, um, that I don't like it if it feels like the place is a mess, Rod always teases me about it. I have certain things and if they're done I feel better. If the washing up's done, if the beds are made, I feel happy. Um, it doesn't matter, there can be two baskets of ironing, folding or anything, but if those basic things are done, I feel happier. (Wendy)

A few mothers reported that having a routine made not only themselves but also their children feel happier as a result:

I think children in general, if they know what's going to happen, they're more happy too. They like schedule. All round you feel good if you can organise some sort of routine, if you want to call it a routine, and I really think the children like it too. (Trish)

Trish felt that because she relied on herself to cope, with no help from her own mother or outside assistance, it reinforced a need within her to be super-organised:

You've just got to use every bit of time in the day the best way you can. Umm, obviously if you've got your mother around [it's easier], but I haven't got my mother around, I've got to be more organised; I've got to do it myself...I think that gets back to what I said before, everything flows, like if you can try to stick to a routine, you're happy, the children are happy, your husband's happy that the house is going smoothly... I mean sure, it won't be perfect and you're going to get problems, but if you can just try and keep things at an even keel.

Cynthia believed that the arrival of her second child heralded the need for greater organisation and self-discipline in order to cope:

I think in one sense, a second child forces you to be more organised. I think in some ways you get a little tighter round the edges, because you have to, and I guess that's good. I think to a certain extent you have to discipline yourself to... like even with kindy, I have to discipline myself to make lunch the night before, and even think about what clothes she's going to wear.

Having a routine was also viewed by mothers in a study by Welles-Nystrom, New, and Richman (1994) as being characteristic of a 'good mother'. Perhaps having a routine to follow or schedule of tasks for the day may assist the mother's organisation and self-discipline. Trish described herself as an organised person, and the term 'self-disciplined' was mentioned frequently in our interviews:

> …it's important to be organised. Like for example, it's tempting to stay in bed in the morning, if no-one's hassling you, it'd be really tempting to stay in bed for an hour or something, but I think, 'No', unless I'm really tired, I'll jump in the shower and then that's out of the way. Because otherwise with that delay, it'll be 2 o'clock or something in the afternoon and you might not have anything done, and I think for me, I just get up and get the day going. I think that's what I'm getting at. And then you'll be happy, because you won't think, 'I'm stressed'.

In her second interview, Trish reiterated this viewpoint:

> …it's good to keep on top of things. You don't just laze around, you've got to get your act together. Get up and think, 'We'll have breakfast at this time-ish', and then try and go out to the park. I think that's how I cope.

However, she also clarified her position by stating she didn't wish to be a Supermum. Trish believed that the schedules and plans of mothers needed to be reasonably flexible as well:

> Only that I don't think the be-all-and-end-all of coping is being super organised. I wouldn't say I was trying to be a Supermum or anything like that and I'm just normal like anyone else but I guess that's my clear struck goal [to be organised]… You've got to keep thinking, 'Well if this isn't working, then ok'. And I'm in a routine, but you can't just think, 'This is *what* I've got to do', you've got to be flexible as well.

To help her be more organised, Wendy writes up goals or lists for each day, but leaves bigger tasks until the weekend when her husband Bill will be home:

> I have a little plan for each day of what I want to get done, um, so that, just their needs come first, for food, or whatever, but in-between their sleep times, I have lists of what I want to get done. I have my little lists of things, 'I'm going to make the bed', 'I'm going to do the washing up and fold the washing', and if I get those things done, I'm happy because they're the day to day things, and anything else that's bigger waits. That's what weekends and evenings are for, the two of us, I find I can handle it. (Wendy)

However, during the focus group discussion, Phillipa stated her disdain at having to frequently organise everyone else in the household. It would be nice she said, if occasionally, someone could organise *her*:

> You've got to be organised. And you've got to organise your husband, and your children and yourself. That's the thing that really bugs me, sometimes I spend all my time organising everyone else, but no-one ever organises me. And that would be really lovely, a real luxury if someone would organise me, I'd love it. Like if someone made decisions for me. An organised husband would help. (laughs)

5.4   Gaining Time-Out

Gaining some space and time away from the normal home routine was recommended by all informants as helping them to cope:

> I think it's just the way we operate as humans to see that sometimes we do need some time-out, to see that this will end, you know, 'Thursday morning I'll have a break', so you can actually see a way out. 'I can do this for a bit longer because I've got a break coming'. I do find exercise to be time-out. My walks really do help. (Cynthia)

> My strategy is that I play sport, and I set aside one night a week for training, and one afternoon on the weekend for playing soccer, so I play that and nothing changes that no matter what else is happening round. I don't care what else is happening around, nothing changes that, that's my time. (Kate)

> I think it's just that stay-at-home thing, get those boring things done and going out and having a bit of fun occasionally, reward yourself. You've got to go out do things with girlfriends who have no children…and I find that little outlet very enjoyable. (Sarah)

Sarah also believed that this time-out to switch off works by keeping her 'sane':

> I make sure I have contact with the outside, with usually other mothers. I try to go for as many walks as I can each week by myself, but that depends on my husband's schedule. It [time-out] keeps you a little bit sane and it keeps you in touch with the world, not somewhere where you have to think constantly of this person on your hip or what they're doing or what they're touching, whatever. It keeps you mentally sound.

Phillipa agreed in that time-out helped her in feeling healthier and in turn being able to cope more effectively:

> If you feel well in yourself and you give yourself time-out, I think that's probably the most important thing, because then you can deal with everything else.

However, taking time-out can sometimes be associated with experiencing guilt or a constant awareness of the child's needs during the time-out activity:

> I'd probably feel guilty [if I was going out and] if I wasn't giving Mitchell my best, I suppose, but I think you need some time to yourself. I go to the gym two to three times a week. (Vanessa)

Kate sometimes experienced guilt, however rationalises that she will be more effective in her role as carer if she benefits from occasional time-out:

> Oh, I get incredibly guilty sometimes. Especially if you have a sick child, whatever, but you also have to think if there's a sick child, there's more demands on your time, they depend on you, and you've got to be mentally healthy, you have to cope. I find it really stressful with the children with little time on my own, and I just find that a healthier me is better for them all over.

Trish described how getting out to meet other mothers helped her to feel less isolated:

> You've got to get out and go pramwalking, or do a sport or get out and about with other mums and have a chat because number one, you're getting out in the fresh air, your child really enjoys it, and everyone's happy. You get out and about and meet other mums, and

getting back to your strategies, that's how you learn that sometimes when you think, 'Wow, I'm doing everything wrong', you speak to someone else and they're even worse than you, so you think, 'I'm not so bad after all'. (laughs)

Trish further explained to me that for her, time-out was related to thinking of one's self, and at the "end of the day", individual happiness was paramount:

I think at the end of the day, if you do what's best for you, and I guess what makes you feel happy and everyone else is happy, then I guess you're doing the right thing. I think you've got to think of yourself too, and if you get too busy thinking about the children and not yourself, it's just natural. I think at the end of the day, if you're not happy, well then the others won't be, because it goes down the line.

5.5 Conclusion

This chapter has revealed the main themes to arise from the series of interviews I held with the mothers associated with how each one said she coped with her day-to-day lifestyle. The mothers coped in three main ways: (a) obtaining outside help, (b) having a plan, and (c) time-out. Help was sought from the mother's own mother and husband. Some degree of help or back-up with tasks was viewed as a great assistance, "having Bill as support certainly makes things a lot easier than they would be otherwise" (Wendy).

However actually being able to ask for assistance was another matter, "I'd feel a bit guilty asking my sister because she's got kids of her own to worry about". Asking for help often induced feelings of awkwardness, obligation or guilt as explained by Cynthia, "people have offered, well the lady up the road, but it's hard, you feel like you're imposing on them", while Sarah said "if you ask friends, you've got to help them back in return…it's just awkward, I don't like to ask people for help".

Having a routine was perceived as an effective coping strategy, "I find routine is how I cope" (Sarah). It also helped to reduce stress as it felt as though tasks were not left neglected or incomplete, "I don't like things hanging over me" (Vanessa). According to Vanessa," when there's an evident routine", she felt like she could cope more effectively. Having a plan helped the mothers feel in greater control of the day's events. "All round you feel good if you can organise some sort of routine, if you want to call it a routine, and I really think the children like it too" (Trish).

A large-scale survey called "Families with Young Children" conducted in the USA, examined the frequency with which parents of young children engage in three representative parenting practices, (a) shared book reading, (b) daily routines (bed, nap, and meal time), and (c) nurturing activities such as hugging and cuddling. It was noted that these three parenting activities, including routines, provided unique opportunities for stimulating cognitive, social, physical, and emotional development in young children. Secondly, only about half of parents with children 1 year or older maintained these daily routines. Younger, lower income, and less-educated parents were less likely to engage in child-rearing activities associated with fostering children's healthy cognitive, social, and emotional development (Britto, Fuligni, & Brooks-Gunn, 2002).

The findings in this chapter also revealed that if the mother didn't take control of the household, there was no-one else mentioned as taking charge or full responsibility. "That's the thing that really bugs me, sometimes I spend all my time organising everyone else, but no-one ever organises me" (Phillipa). So having a routine may be a nurturing and healthy practice for the mothers to engage in for the well-being of their children. It may help them to feel like they're coping more effectively.

But who nurtures the mothers, or cares for the carer? Everyone needs to feel valued, loved and regardless of appearance, behaviour, or level of achievement. Perhaps that's why mothers as parents also need to be parented for a while too. Blohm (2001) conducted a phenomenological study of the experience of being nurtured as an adult. According to Blohm (2001), being nurtured as an adult involves a felt sense of 'taking in'. Feeling nurtured leads to well-being. This personal change generates an enhanced sense of self. One of the essential qualities recognised as being part of feeling nurtured as an adult included a recognition of a personal need, and being given time by someone or something. Nurturing requires time. So it only makes sense that if the mother needs a break from all of her nurturing of other family members and needs to nurture herself, she needs time-*out* from her role, and time to herself (Blohm, 2001).

All informants recommended gaining some space and time away from the normal home routine as a strategy that helped them to cope. Time-out was seen as a way of coping because it offered a break and reward needed to maintain mental health and also a chance to catch up with friends. Methods of achieving time-out included physical activity, such as gym or walks or going out with friends. Time-out decreased any sense of isolation and after talking to other mothers about their problems, the mothers often discovered that their situations or coping strategies weren't such a 'failure' after all. Despite experiencing guilt at taking time-out, 'at the end of the day', an individual's happiness was viewed as paramount, "I think you've got to think of yourself too...I think at the end of the day, if you're not happy, well then the others won't be" (Trish).

Chapter 6 discusses the main findings in the context of the wider research literature. It helps more closely examine how mothers cope and maintain perceptions of subjective wellness.

References

Bennett, E. A. (1981). Coping in the puerperium: The reported experience of new mothers. *Journal of Psychosomatic Research, 25,* 13–21.

Blohm, L. L. (2001). The experience of being nurtured as an adult. *Dissertation Abstracts International, 62,* (4-B), 2047.

Britto, P. R., Fuligni, A. S., & Brooks-Gunn, J. (2002). Reading, rhymes, and routines: American parents and their young children. In N. Halfon, & K. T. McLearn (Eds.), *Child rearing in America:*

Challenges facing parents with young children (pp. 117–145). New York: Cambridge University Press.

Carpentier, N., & White, D. (2002). Cohesion of the primary social network and sustained service use before the first psychiatric hospitalisation. *Journal of Behavioral Health Services & Research, 29,* 404–418.

Dardis, R., Derrick, F., Lehfeld, A., & Wolfe, K. E. (1981). Cross-section studies of recreation expenditures in 1981 in the US. *Journal of Leisure Research, 13,* 181–194.

De Nooijer, J., Lechner, L., & De Vries, H. (2001). Help-seeking behaviour for cancer symptoms: Perceptions of patients and general practitioners. *Psycho-Oncology, 10,* 469–478.

Dunkel-Schetter, C., Blasband, D., Feinstein, L. G., & Bennett Herbert, T. (1992). Elements of supportive interactions: When are attempts to help effective? In S. Spacapan & S. Oskamp (Eds.), *Helping and being helped in the real world* (pp. 83–114). Newbury Park, CA: Sage Publications.

Fang, S. -R. S., & Frizzell, T. (1998). The impact of a parent education program during mothers' and fathers' transitions to parenthood. *ERIC Document,* AN, ED433153.

Feeney, J. A. (2002). Early parenting and parental attachment: Links with offspring's attachment and perceptions of social support. *Journal of Family Studies, 8,* 5–23.

Henderson, K. A., Bialeschki, M. D., Shaw S. M., & Freysinger, V. J. (1989). *A Leisure of one's own: A feminist perspective on women's leisure.* PA., USA: Venture.

Kahn, R. L. (1979). Aging and social support. In M. W. Riley (Ed.), *Aging from birth to death: Interdisciplinary perspectives* (pp. 77–91). Boulder, Colorado: Westview.

Krauss, K., & Wyngaarden, M. (1993). The Impact of parent groups on mothers of infants with disabilities. *Journal of Early Intervention, 17,* 8–20.

Peters, F. P. M. L., & Bayer, H. (1999). 'No-show' for initial screening at a community mental health centre: Rate, reasons, and further help-seeking. *Social Psychiatry and Psychiatric Epidemiology, 34,* 323–327.

Reifman, A., & Dunkel-Schetter, C. (1990). Stress, structural social support, and well-being in university students. *American Journal of College Health, 38,* 271–277.

Rhodes, J. (1982). Unemployment and leisure. In S. A. Glyptis (Ed.), *Prospects for leisure and work. Proceedings of Regional Seminars. Leisure Studies Association Conference Papers, 12,* pp. 99–101.

Tarkka, M.-T., Paunonen, M., & Laippala, P. (1996). Social support provided by nurses to recent mothers on a maternity ward. *Journal of Advanced Nursing, 23,* 1202–1206.

Welles-Nystrom, B., New, R., & Richman, A. (1994). The 'good mother': A comparative study of Swedish, Italian and American maternal behavior and goals. *Scandinavian Journal of Caring Sciences, 8,* 81–86.

Chapter 6
Towards a Positive Model of Coping

*We've tried lots of strategies, some have worked, yes, it's been
fantastic, so I have felt more confident, felt like I've got
strategies that work, felt like I know my babies well enough to do
what's right for them, and um, what I do works, so I felt good. A
lot of it is really just responsive to what's going on, so if things
are on a cycle where they're not going as well, then that's gonna
make me feel less assured and less confident* (Wendy).

Abstract To cope and manage motherhood feels good. It leads to a sense of satisfaction and being in control. Mothers are aware of more effective or higher levels
of coping as they felt less stressed as a result and could cruise along and feel more
enjoyment with their role. All of the informants identified with the 'Coping Cycle'
where they developed skill, confidence and a sense of hardiness through a process
of attempts and trials of coping strategies. As motherhood constantly throws daily
challenges, it is important to persist with the Cycle and build resilience as it will
increase individual sense of control and subjective well-being.

6.1 Introduction

Coping includes efforts to manage stressful, challenging or difficult events. Similarly,
all of the mothers providing personal stories for this book agreed that on a day-to-day
basis, mothering was difficult. It requires energy, attention and use of strategies in
order to cope. This chapter further examines mothers' preferred coping strategies
and contains a discussion of the major findings and considers their implications in
terms of the related literature.

© The Author(s) 2018
J. L. Currie, *Managing Motherhood*, SpringerBriefs in Well-Being and Quality
of Life Research, https://doi.org/10.1007/978-981-13-0338-8_6

6.2   The Meaning of Coping in the Context of the Daily Lifestyles of Mothers

For the mothers I interviewed, the concept of coping was ultimately equated with acceptance of a socially constructed image of the 'coping mother'. On the one hand, completing tasks led to a feeling of satisfaction, of being on top of things and a good household manager. However, this meant that the mothers were surveilling their own task performance. Effective coping and 'household management' mattered a great deal to them. This feature may have also related to the concept of the mothers perceiving different levels of coping.

Mothers identified effective or *higher levels* of coping when:

- strategies were perceived as being successfully implemented,
- perceived stress levels were reduced,
- confidence levels were at their highest, and
- satisfaction and enjoyment levels related to the mothering role in general were also at their highest.

Therefore, gaining a sense of coping enhances the mother's satisfaction in her role.

While coping was related to a mother feeling as if she was *getting things done* and functioning well in her role, at the same time, an element of *quality, enjoyment and realism* was still desired. This was preferable to the mother completing all tasks but experiencing a sense of drudgery. This theme highlighted the mothers' acknowledgement of the importance of gaining subjective wellness.

For this group of mothers, coping was also related to greater feelings of *being in control of one's situation,* or an increased internal locus of control. People with an internal locus of control are characterised by their belief that what happens to them is a consequence of their own actions and is within their control (Duff, 1997, p. 5). Control relates to hardiness or how well an individual handles stress or demands placed upon her (Naughton, 1997). The findings suggest that mothers who cope also exhibit a degree of hardiness.

According to the mothers, 'just scraping through' was synonymous with low-level coping. This finding may be interpreted as the mothers justifying any perceived poor coping outcomes. Rather than admit to outright failure, the mothers may have been attempting to save face, so they didn't feel ashamed or inadequate. Alternatively, they may have wished to legitimise their efforts and recognise that an outcome at any level is 'ok'.

When analysing what the mothers needed to cope *with*, the main themes to emerge related to key ideas around the mothers' philosophy of mothering. There appears to be a strong perception among these women that social pressure is high and they willingly/unwillingly strive to fit the ideal, or justify why they can't. The next section discusses the challenges mothers had to cope with on a daily basis.

6.3 The Situations and Demands Mothers Cope With

6.3.1 Changed Lifestyle

All informants noted that they had to deal with a change in lifestyle since the baby was born. It was referred to as a "shock". Lack of freedom and being on call 24 hours a day were noted as examples of this phenomena. The transition period in new motherhood can be associated with a changed self identity, reduced freedom and levels of tiredness never experienced before. As Schmied and Everitt (1996, p. 114) described; "It was like walking into someone else's life, this was not my life anymore". Additionally, typical lifestyle changes may be experienced differently by individual mothers. According to Tarkka, Paunonen, and Laippala (1996, p. 117), the main lifestyle changes new mothers often experience include mental and social ones such as increased isolation and role restrictions. The new mother acquires an overwhelmingly new identity, and also encounters the following lifestyle 'losses':

- body changes, such as weight gain
- loss of independence, for example giving up paid work
- increased isolation, for instance lack of adult interaction.

  Research conducted by Walker and Wilging (2000) discovered that mothers had to deal with stress caused by:

- the transition or changes experienced by mothers in their new role and lifestyle
- retained postnatal weight
- lack of social support.

Through her struggle to integrate her new mothering role into her personal identity, a mother may experience depressed mood. Depressed symptoms may impact negatively on coping (Maushart, 1997). However, no informants participating in the research for this book identified as feeling depressed or unwell.

  It is interesting to note previous studies revealing that mothers perceiving minimal personal lifestyle changes as a result of the birth of a child experience the greatest satisfaction with the new mothering role (Schmied & Everitt, 1996, p. 123). Care of younger babies under 6 months may also feel more constraining than care of older children. Schmied and Everitt (1996) reported the period immediately following birth being associated with the least amount of time to self or for self-care, an increase in role conflict and experience of physical illnesses. This feature may have asserted the greatest impact on Trish, Vanessa and Wendy with their very young babies.

6.3.2   Difficulty of the Mothering Role with Lack of Social Recognition

The literature has reported incongruence between what health professionals such as nurses believe is important and essential to coping with the mothering role, compared with the views of mothers themselves. Midwives have traditionally emphasised the medical, biological and 'mothercraft' aspects of motherhood focusing on care of the baby, while mothers have expressed they essentially want to feel as though they are coping.

Women often feel totally unprepared for the challenges associated with the mothering role (Schmied & Everitt, 1996, p. 114). Mothers have stated that they want information on the social and emotional experience of motherhood, how to balance the demands of all family members, plus find some time for self. Vehvilainen-Julkunen (1995) found that mothers expressed quite strongly that the ability to cope with day-to-day situations is an extremely important topic that they wished to have more information about.

Similar to the findings contained in Harris' (1998) and Wearing's (1984) studies, my informants may have experienced stress because they identified themselves as having primary responsibility for childcare. Role strain is the perceived difficulty in achieving role obligations. It is related to negative psychological and physical effects (Seib & Muller, 1999). According to Seib and Miller (1999) and Wanamaker and Bird (1990), even though some employed mothers experience more role strain than non-employed mothers, they often experience less depression and anxiety due to improved self-esteem, financial status and social support obtainable through paid work. The mothers in this book were not currently obtaining esteem or financial rewards from involvement in outside employment.

For the mothers who felt they were coping adequately, my findings revealed a current of dissatisfaction or a wanting by the mothers to be recognised for a job well done. I gained a sense that the mothers felt that their roles were not being socially recognised as important. For example, the findings revealed a sense of social obligation by Cynthia to her family and outside community. However, I believe she also would have liked some social recognition of her independent contributions and volunteering in the community.

Coping, especially for women, is affected by gender roles. According to Duxbury, Higgins, and Lee (1994), Raskin, Kummel, and Bannister (1998) and Schmied and Everitt (1996), family roles are considered more central to women than men and are also potentially a greater source of concern or stress. Mothers are often concerned with being a 'good mother'. They tend to place emphasis on the social and gender perspectives of the mothering role (Schmied & Everitt, 1996; Vehvilainen-Julkunen, 1995). Therefore, they may equate successful coping with having achieved a higher level of femininity, or a more positive and fulfilled state of who she is striving to be.

6.3.3 The Image of the Coping Mother

While everyday coping efforts may not be widely recognised by the community, there is pressure exerted from institutions for mothers to succeed. Parenting is not something we adequately prepare people for in a practical or emotional manner. It is acknowledged as difficult, but at the end of the day, there is public expectation that parents *will* succeed (Parenting South Australia, 2010).

Harris (1998) found that the mothers' choice of childcare coping strategies were linked to the values they had about mothering. These values were highly influenced by the mothers' notions of what society considered a good mother to be. Similarly for my book, the mothers' values about 'good' mothering were socially influenced and provided the context in which strategies were selected or discarded. The attributes of a good mother identified by Harris (1998) and Wearing (1984), included patience, love, support, selfless availability, respect, being there for the children, positive interaction with the children, controlling your own anger and being non-judgemental.

All mothers were aware of social pressures to cope well in their role as mother. The mothers' acknowledgement of the importance of physical, social and emotional well-being in coping revealed their acceptance of a socially constructed image of the coping mother. There appeared to be a perception among these women that social pressure is high. They willingly or unwillingly strived to fulfil the ideal, or justify why they couldn't. This finding concurs with that of Dix (1987) and Schmied and Everitt (1996), in that mothers like to feel as though they are coping. Mothers are concerned with being a 'good' mother. In addition, many mothers in Rowe, Temple, and Hawthorne's (1996, p. S56) study described difficulties or perceived barriers in attending community groups for improving their parenting skills. They felt there was a social stigma attached to mothers participating in meetings addressing emotional or other problems.

All of the informants participating in interviews for this book individually identified as feeling well. However, they too may have been aware of a social stigma attached with admitting to not coping and needing help. They may have not felt comfortable disclosing to the researcher any overwhelming stress, personal emotional problems or issues surrounding not coping effectively. Any perception by the informants that they 'needed to cope', or at least provide this impression, may have been a factor driving their responses. Many mothers keep up a façade of 'I'm coping', because that's what 'good' mothers do (Dix, 1987).

Mothers who feel as though they are coping can put aside feelings of awkwardness when seeking help and assistance. It is a shame that in westernised cultures we have often lost much in the way of community connectedness, close neighbours, and the wonderful support able to be gained from extended families who like to help each other.

Exhibiting signs of severe tiredness or depression is taboo. It creates the impression a mother is not coping in her role. Learned coping, or culturally expected coping may pressure mothers into feeling they should 'get over it', or try harder to cope (Crouch & Manderson, 1993, p. 159). It is perhaps due to this reason that previous studies have reported mothers faking that they are coping or pretending to be enjoying the motherhood experience (Levine, 1990; Maushart, 1997). Attempting to have others believe she is coping by 'faking it', through putting up a stoic façade or cool appearance, may help a mother experience a sense of social acceptance and approval. However underneath, the mother may still feel stressed, exhausted or frustrated. Losing one's cool while a child has a tantrum in a shopping mall, having an untidy house or appearance, or interacting in a depressed manner, are not deemed to be socially acceptable behaviours in today's success-driven society.

Future research could further explore the notion of 'real' mothering, where stress, tiredness and lack of coping or sense of control at times are exposed as normal experiences. It would be helpful to examine the relationship between self esteem, the amount of perceived external approval and social recognition received, and feelings of internal satisfaction and success in one's mothering role.

Raskin, Kummel, and Bannister (1998) concluded that it is perfectly normal for mothers to feel tired, or down at times. Nevertheless, it is healthy for mothers to find ways to manage or master day-to-day situations. Feeling in control by implementing effective coping strategies will decrease the risk of chronic stress. The next section will discuss the strategies mothers of young children used in order to cope with their day-to-day lifestyles.

6.4   Strategies Mothers Use to Cope with Their Daily Lifestyles

6.4.1   Outside Help

Pridham (1997) categorised three types of social support:

1. emotional support: concern understanding, encouragement
2. informational support: advice to aid in problem solving
3. instrumental support: practical aid with tasks, contribution of resources.

Instrumental support was frequently mentioned by my informants as being the most highly valued form of assistance, and yet it seemed to be the most difficult type to ask for or accept. It had the potential to be highly intrusive if externally sourced. Mothers who had their own mothers nearby felt they could access this form of assistance to gain some time-out or minor cleaning help. Other examples included taking turns with other mothers in babysitting, or accepting help from friends. However, these strategies were not used very frequently. Mothers were highly aware of inconveniencing the other party or of the reciprocal obligation to offer some sort of comparable help in return.

The informants exhibited a capable and independent approach to the care of the family and household. They tended to cope on their own with little help from others. Perhaps there is more freedom, independence and control involved in 'doing it on your own'. The findings showed that in the situation where support was to be used, it would only be taken up when it was deemed to be relatively unobtrusive, undemanding, and able to be readily reciprocated. 'Outside help' was most likely to be of a nature involving the least amount of 'reciprocal obligation'. That is, a mother would pay for childcare or cleaning as she saw it as involving little or no return obligation. It was considered to be less complicated and not implicating the mother into feeling as though she should perform some sort of gesture in return.

This finding supports the research conducted by d'Abbs (1991) and Harris (1998) who found that mothers were more likely to employ coping strategies engaging the least amount of reciprocal obligation. This strategy also reflects the nature of the prime responsibility accepted by most mothers for childcare and the running of their households. The group of mothers in this study attempted to manage their own home situation primarily by themselves. However, in the event that outside help was deemed necessary in order to cope effectively, the mothers often described their personal struggle or real difficulties in accepting assistance. Limited assistance from one's own mother was deemed acceptable and those with mothers available and living nearby were able to access cleaning and child minding assistance more readily. The mothers who didn't have their own mother living nearby or available to readily assist them seemed to lament the apparent lack of support. They revealed additional efforts were individually expended, drawing on even greater personal strengths to cope on their own.

The barriers to accessing outside assistance or support seem to hinge greatly on ideological beliefs about the extent of the selflessness expected of mothers, employed or working in the home. Australian Institute of Family Studies statistics (Higgins & Morse, 2000; Kolar & Soriano, 2000) show most Australians believe both parents should share the physical and emotional care of their children as well as their economic support. However, studies show that ultimately the mother is primary caregiver in the domestic sphere of both dual and single-income families (Donath, 2000; Reid-Boyd, 2000). Even the increase in women's labour market participation over the past 40 years has also occurred without any corresponding revolution in the care of children at home. Women wanting more symmetrical household arrangements tend to rely on paid childcare, or for the less wealthy, grandparents. In reality, childcare is not undertaken as a dual role by both parents.

Examples of emotional support accessed by the mothers included Wendy talking to her husband, or to her friend who is also a mother of twins and understood what she was going through. The mothers in Tarkka et al. (1996) study found that emotional support, principally from husbands was the most effective form of support mentioned by the mothers. In this study, the mothers mentioned examples of informational support such as telephone help lines, community nurses, or talking to other mothers in order to compare situations. The public health nurses in Tarkka et al. (1996) study were viewed by mothers as providing a competent source of information, affirmation and support. This particular type of support was positively correlated with a mother's ability to cope with childcare.

A satisfactory amount of support received can positively affect the coping experiences of new mothers (Schmied & Everitt, 1996). For example, social support can be especially helpful to the new mother when she is attempting to adapt to this major life change (Pridham, 1997). The negative effect of stressors, or the external demands mothers cope with, may be buffered or reduced by the availability of resources or instrumental support, and informational support (d'Abbs, 1991). Reciprocity of support provided between parents and other groups of people outside the household is influenced by family income and level of parental education.

Other factors predicting supportive parental behaviours include degree of parental warmth, monitoring, and supportive behaviours, such as 'telling others positive things about the child' and not 'sparing the hug' (Hsu, 2002). A higher degree of financial strain in a family can predict lower quantities of parental monitoring, however, the less the family financial strain is, the higher the parental monitoring is. Significantly, according to Hsu (2002), the higher degree of supportive parental behaviours, the higher is the child's resulting self-esteem.

Other recent studies of the attitudes of parents of young children have found a contradiction in that on the one hand, both parents agree that women are expected to return to paid work after having children. On the other hand, nearly all women surveyed felt that mothers should provide all the care for their young children (Probert, 2001). Even as far back as the '70 s, Pybus, Brennan, Gillan, Rayner, and Scott (1978, p. 35) recommended that the care of the baby be given a different name to 'mothering', as it denoted the female gender as the prime carer, and father as 'helper'; "In focusing on the mother as caregiver we are neglecting the definite contribution of the father…".

Further studies show that mothers would appreciate a greater contribution from fathers in the caregiving role. The mothers in a study by Milkie, Bianchi, Mattingly, and Robinson (2002) perceived much less father involvement in actual parenting than fathers perceived, especially in disciplining and providing emotional support for their children. The discrepancies between mothers' and fathers' perception of ideal compared with actual parenting levels were related to well-being. If fathers were seen as less than ideally involved in nurturant parenting, parents, including mothers, reported more stress. For example, according to Milkie et al. (2002) less than ideal father involvement in disciplining children was associated with mothers' higher stress levels. Additionally, the discrepancy in mothers' expectations about father involvement in play and monitoring children was correlated with mothers' increased feelings of unfairness in the household division of labour.

However, Mulsow, Caldera, Pursley, Reifman, and Huston (2002) found that a mother's personality was most predictive of parenting stress in a study of 134 mothers and their infants at ages 1, 6, 15, 24, and 36 months, cross-sectionally and longitudinally. Intimacy with partner reduced parenting stress early in the infant's life and at 36 months, whereas general social support was more important in the second year. Child temperament was influential at 1 and 36 months. Unfortunately, a psychological account of personality styles or types was not included in the present study, however, child's temperament was noted by the mothers as being an influential factor in their coping experience.

My findings reveal an expressed need by mothers for basic social support by peers. The mothers felt that interacting with other mothers might help them cope better. My group of informants only included women of Anglo Saxon background. Coping strategies employed by women of varying ethnic heritage could differ, such as being more likely to involve relatives or an extended family in the caring role (Kobus & Reyes, 2000).

Harris (1998) concluded that it was legitimate for a woman to provide support, but not to accept it herself. If a mother can manage the situation on her own, she will. If she cannot, she will choose strategies that engage the least reciprocal obligation (d'Abbs, 1991; Harris, 1998). These studies reflect the lived experience of Phillipa who said:

> But I think one of the more personal things is being able to ask for help. And that, I would say, is a problem that I have, is that I don't ask. I'd be comfortable to ask my mum, husband or dad or sister, but outside of that, even when it's offered, I find it hard to accept it. (Phillipa)

Andrykowski et al. (2002) stated that individuals also differ with regard to informational coping style, that is, the extent to which and manner in which they seek health-relevant information and respond to threatening events. Individuals characterised by a 'monitoring' coping style (*monitors*) tend to actively scan the environment for health-relevant information that may help coping outcomes. Those characterized by a 'blunting' style (*blunters*) tend to avoid or minimise health-relevant information. Under conditions of low threat, monitors and blunters do not differ much with regard to cognition, affect, or behaviour. However, when confronted with a threatening health event, such as a breast biopsy or a very sick child, differences emerge. Monitors are likely to respond with distress because of their tendency to actively seek information and to amplify threat both cognitively and emotionally. Blunters are less likely to evidence distress because they tend to avoid and blunt threatening health information.

6.4.2 Routine

Having a scheduled plan or routine was perceived by all informants to be an effective coping strategy. It helped the mothers to feel as though tasks were not left incomplete. This related directly to the notion of 'what is coping?' because for the mothers this meant 'getting things done'. Therefore a 'routinised' existence was often described as assisting with coping ability as you were more likely to effectively manage your workload and have a plan.

A routinised lifestyle may be more preventive in terms of stress than having to learn to cope with unexpected pressures. If a mother can manage external events to a degree or keep them as routine as possible, highly developed coping skills will not normally be necessary (Bruess & Richardson, 1989, p. 56).

6.4.3   Time-Out

Finding time-out for self, without experiencing any associated guilt, can be a valuable way of reducing stress and tension, and of restoring some personal identity or lowered self-esteem (Currie, 2018; Littlewood & McHugh, 1997). A mother should be supported and encouraged to attend to her own health and well-being. The increased awareness and acting on of the rights of mothers to achieve some sort of balance in their roles could be due to internalising a new socially constructed notion of health, or rights of the individual. To be healthiest, mothers must let go of the notion of being a Supermum because it is unrealistic and we can't be perfect. These kinds of 'new age' media messages may appear as radical to some mothers, but they may help others to feel justified or vindicated in attempting to take time-out from the caring role. According to Dix (1987, pp. 204–205), mothers are vulnerable to the 'guilt trap', but taking time-out can help. It was advised to help avoid the potential triggers of Postnatal Depression.

A mother's health level is related to her experiencing the subjective wellness associated with coping (Tarkka et al., 1996). My findings revealed a desire by the mothers to achieve a balance between completing household chores, outside responsibilities providing attention for children or other family members, and achieving some time-out or reward for self. Schmied and Everitt (1996, p. 111) found that especially during the postnatal period, women want to be able to access greater information on how to balance the demands of babies, husbands or partners, and to also find some time out for themselves.

6.5   The Coping Cycle

The research methodology of grounded theory includes the development and evolution of conceptual models emerging from the data as the study unfolds. The findings presented in this book support the notion that having an effective array of strategies available to implement as a challenging situation arises, may lead to greater hardiness or a feeling of being able to take on further challenges readily and confidently. A theoretical illustration of this cycle of coping is illustrated in Fig. 6.1. The experience of at least having been through the cycle once, or having tried strategies before, means that mothers can face future situations with greater confidence.

All the informants stated to me that they identified with the coping cycle diagram. Wendy said, "I really identified with it when I saw it". If a mother felt like her coping strategy worked, she felt more confident as a result. The feelings gained from coming out of the cycle were also described in terms of subjective wellness. The cycle was used as a training ground for trialing new strategies and approaches to situations. Furthermore, when facing new challenges, mothers could draw upon the courage and confidence built up from having succeeded the cycle previously:

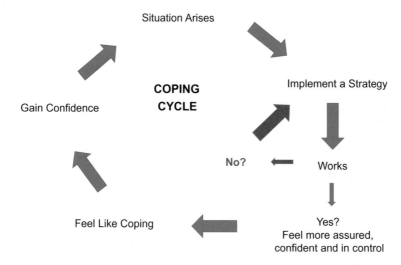

Fig. 6.1 The coping cycle

When you are dealing with something new and different you'll have to use the same cycle to bring yourself back to feeling more confident and again know that you can again deal with this new stage of your child's development, like you did the last stage. The only advantage is that you've coped with things before, coped with the stages before, so that [having been through the cycle] is a source of confidence, that you will get there with time and patience. (Wendy)

6.6   Conclusion

According to Aldwin (1994), the origin of stress lies within the environment. The informants have generally described their own environments as busy and challenging, but as also causing their stress. However, each mother was able to nominate a method in which she attempted to deal with a stressful situation. A self-perception of dealing effectively with a situation, pressure or scenario was described as making her feel as though she was coping.

Figure 6.1 identifies the confidence and sense of resilience gained from being able to continually handle a situation with an effective coping strategy. Once a mother has faced a similar problem and moved through the cycle a few times, she can feel more in control and in a position to know what to expect, and do, on the next occasion. This strength-building is conceptualised as an increased sense of resilience. "Resilience is a person's ability to cope with living in spite of stresses. It's about coping with problems, and building strengths that protect and promote well-being" (Parenting SA, 2010).

Chapter 7 clarifies the conditions or factors noted by the informants as limiting or enhancing coping success, and either making it easier or more difficult to cope.

References

Aldwin, C. (1994). *Stress, coping, and development: An integrative perspective.* New York: Guilford.

Andrykowski, M. A., Carpenter, J. S., Studts, J. L., Cordova, M. J., Cunningham, L. C., Beacham, A., et al. (2002). Psychological impact of benign breast biopsy: A longitudinal, comparative study. *Health Psychology, 21,* 485–494.

Bruess, C., & Richardson, G. (1989). *Decisions for health* (3rd ed.). Dubuque, Iowa: WM C. Brown.

Crouch, M., & Manderson, L. (1993). *New motherhood. Cultural and personal transitions in the 1980s.* Camberwell, Victoria: Gordon & Breach.

Currie, J. L. (2018). *Radical leisure. How mothers gain well-being and control through participation in exercise classes.* Champaign, IL.: Common Ground Research Networks.

d'Abbs, P. (1991). *Who helps? Support networks and social policy in Australia. Australian Institute of Family Studies, Monograph No. 12.* Melbourne: Australian Institute of Family Studies.

Dix, C. (1987). *The new mother syndrome. Coping with postnatal stress and depression.* North Sydney: Allen and Unwin.

Donath, S. (2000, July). *Pipe and slippers or kitchen sink? Coming home from work.* Paper presented at family futures: Issues in research and policy, 7th Australian Institute of Family Studies Conference, Sydney.

Duff, J. (1997). *Repressive denial, locus of control, and coping styles, and their relationships with immunosuppression, cardiovascular function and health outcomes.* Retrieved from http://www.adhd.com.au/immunity.html.

Duxbury, L., Higgins, C., & Lee, C. (1994). Work-family conflict: A comparison by gender, family type, and perceived control. *Journal of Family Issues, 15,* 449–466.

Harris, N. (1998). Coping with young children: How do mothers do it? *Proceedings of the 6th Australian Institute of Family Studies (AIFS) Conference* (pp. 1–5). Melbourne: AIFS.

Higgins, S., & Morse, C. (2000, July). *Combining Parenting and Paid Work: Sharing child care in dual income families.* Paper presented at Family Futures: Issues in research and policy, 7th Australian Institute of Family Studies Conference, Sydney.

Hsu, S. -Y. (2002). Social capital, parental behaviors and children's self-esteem in the family context. *Dissertation Abstracts International, 62,* 4348-A.

Kobus, K., & Reyes, O. (2000). A descriptive study of urban Mexican American adolescents' perceived stress and coping. *Hispanic Journal of Behavioral Science, 22,* 163–178.

Kolar, V., & Soriano, G. (2000). *Parenting in Australian families. A comparative study of Anglo, Torres Strait Islander and Vietnamese families. Research Report No. 5. Australian Institute of Family Studies.* Melbourne: Australian Institute of Family Studies.

Levine, K. (1990). *Coping with stress. Parents, 6,* 68–70.

Littlewood, J., & McHugh, N. (1997). *Maternal distress and postnatal depression. The myth of madonna.* Basingstoke, UK: Macmillan.

Maushart, S. (1997). *The mask of motherhood. How motherhood changes everything and why we pretend it doesn't.* Milson's Point, Sydney: Random House.

Milkie, M. A., Bianchi, S. M., Mattingly, M. J., & Robinson, J. P. (2002). Gendered Division of Childrearing: Ideals, Realities, and the Relationship to Parental Well-Being. *Sex Roles, 47,* 21–38.

Mulsow, M., Caldera, Y. M., Pursley, M., Reifman, A., & Huston, A. C. (2002). Multilevel factors influencing maternal stress during the first three years. *Journal of Marriage & the Family, 64,* 944–956.

Naughton, F. O. (1997). *Stress and coping.* Northridge, USA: California State University. Retrieved from http://www.csu.edu/~vcpsy00h/students/coping.htm.

Parenting South Australia (SA). (2010). *Coping Skills. Resilience. Parent Easy Guide 18.* Adelaide: Children, Youth and Women's Health Service, Department of Health, Government of South Australia.

Pridham, K. F. (1997). Mother's help-seeking as care initiated in a social context. *Image—the Journal of Nursing Scholarship, 29,* 65–70.

Probert, B. (2001). 'Grateful slaves' or 'self-made women': A matter of choice or policy? *Redress, 11,* 2–11.

Pybus, M., Brennan, M., Gillan, B., Rayner, L., & Scott, B. (1978). *A longitudinal study of new mothers: A student exercise.* Palmerston, New Zealand: Massey University.

Raskin, P. M., Kummel, P., & Bannister, T. (1998). The relationship between coping styles, attachment, and career salience in partnered working women with children. *Journal of Career Assessment, 6,* 403–416.

Reid-Boyd, E. (2000, July). *Being There: Mothers who stay at home.* Paper presented at the 7th Australian Institute of Family Studies Conference, Sydney.

Rowe, L., Temple, S., & Hawthorne, G. (1996). Mothers' emotional needs and difficulties after childbirth. *Clinical Psychologist, 25,* S53–S58.

Seib, B., & Muller, J. (1999). The effect of different work schedules on role strain of Australian working mothers: A pilot study. *Journal of Applied Health Behaviour, 1,* 9–15.

Schmied, V., & Everitt, L. (1996). Postnatal care: Poor cousin or priority area? In L. Barclay & L. Jones (Eds.), *Midwifery: Trends in clinical practice* (pp. 107–126). South Melbourne: Churchill Livingstone.

Tarkka, M.-T., Paunonen, M., & Laippala, P. (1996). Social support provided by nurses to recent mothers on a maternity ward. *Journal of Advanced Nursing, 23,* 1202–1206.

Vehvilainen-Julkunen, K. (1995). Health promotion in families with newborn children at home: Clients' views. *Social Sciences in Health: International Journal of Research & Practice, 1,* 3–13.

Walker, L., & Wilging, S. (2000). Rediscovering the "M" in "MCH": Maternal health promotion after childbirth. *Journal of Obstetric, Gynaecologic and Neonatal Nursing, 29,* 229–236.

Wannamaker, N. J., & Bird, G. W. (1990). Coping with stress in dual-career marriages. *International Journal of Sociology of the Family, 20,* 199–212.

Wearing, B. (1984). *The ideology of motherhood.* Sydney: George Allen and Unwin.

Chapter 7
Conditions Affecting Coping

Abstract The cycle of coping introduced in Chap. 6 can be affected by numerous unexpected factors or additional conditions. According to the mothers, the longer you have been a mother makes it easier to cope, plus it requires an element of persistence and tenacity. However, coping will be influenced by the context of the situation and environment, such as the presence of a sick child, or children growing older. Ultimately, the mother's coping experience was highly influenced by her obligation to the happiness and welfare of her children; "If they're happy, you're happy". Learning to cope may be compared to the stages of learning a motor skill model used in explaining the acquisition of skills in sport. The highest skill level is characterised by confidence, efficiency, a fluid and consistent approach to tasks, and the ability to detect and correct one's own errors.

7.1 Introduction

According to the World Health Organisation (2014), mental health is defined as a state of well-being in which every individual realises his or her own potential, can cope with the normal stresses of life, can work productively and fruitfully, and is able to make a contribution to her or his community." Therefore if a mother can cope more effectively with her everyday lifestyle, she will promote her own sense of mental well-being and overall health. Coping enhances a mother's ability to function and contribute meaningfully in daily life—but to also be in a place where she can relax—be able to cruise along at a more enjoyable and manageable level.

The discussion contained in Chap. 6 outlined a cycle of coping scenario illustrating how a mother grows in overall resilience and confidence. As part of that process, the learning involved takes time and practice. As a mother moves from being beginner status, such as with the arrival of her first baby, to being highly skilled and experienced, she progresses through distinct, although continuous, stages. She will refine her coping strategy's execution, and modify it where necessary. As she gains

J. L. Currie, *Managing Motherhood*, SpringerBriefs in Well-Being and Quality of Life Research, https://doi.org/10.1007/978-981-13-0338-8_7

in overall coping ability, confidence and feelings of competence, a mother is now capable of detecting errors in execution of coping strategies and more adaptable to changing environmental conditions.

However, an analysis of the major findings reveals certain conditions that may affect the cycle of coping. Chapter 7 clarifies those conditions or factors noted by the informants as limiting or enhancing coping success. These factors either made it easier or more difficult to cope. The following sections include an explanation of the meaning of context, the impact of the ever-changing and evolving strategies a mother is faced with, the effect of children on coping, and other conditions nominated by the mothers.

7.2   What Factors Can Make It Harder or Easier to Cope?

7.2.1   The Longer You Have Been a Mother Can Make It Easier to Cope

Sometimes knowing which strategy to implement was related to perceiving an enhancement in skill and experience gained from having subsequent children, "I think knowing what to do can also vary with time, I think the longer you've been a mother then that can make it [coping] easier" (Wendy), or "I don't worry about Adam as much as I used to worry about Mitchell" (Vanessa). Trish further explained this phenomenon or the perceived difference in coping with a second baby compared with the first:

> Yeah, because you know what to expect and they give you a little cry and you sort of think, 'Oh well, they're not going to die', and you don't rush into the room. It's been much easier than with the first one. Yeah, I think the first child, you're so wiped out and blown away by the whole thing and so tired and the second time I didn't feel so tired, I guess because you know what to expect.

It is interesting to note from observational research carried out by Kaitz et al. (2000) that mothers of subsequent babies were no more effective at soothing a newborn baby's cry than first-time mothers. Effective coping may be strongly related to confidence gained from subjective personal perceptions of being an experienced mother and exposure to practice.

This factor may also relate to a positive evaluation of one's own mothering ability or level of self-esteem. Self-esteem is an important determinant of a mother's coping and feelings of control. Rowe, Temple, and Hawthorne (1996) and Tarkka, Paunonen, & Laippala (1996) found a strong correlation between a mother's self concept and her coping. Self-esteem may be positively affected by how successful we view our coping efforts to be. For this group of mothers, perceived levels of coping effectiveness affected how well they perceived themselves to be performing overall as a mother. In this study, perceptions of coping may have been positively affected by those mothers who had high levels of trait, or personality-based self-esteem. Mothers with higher self-esteem would be buffered during stressful events by having a more confident, and positive outlook towards tasks to be accomplished. A positive and confident self-image positively affects how well a mother feels she is succeeding in childcare and how well she is able to respond to a child's needs (Mercer, 1995; Tarkka et al., 1996; Younger, 1991).

Sethi (1995) purported that it can often be harder for first time mothers with young babies to cope. In this study, some mothers pointed out that their second baby was easier to handle due to growth in personal awareness and confidence in general handling skills. A second child allows for greater exposure to practice. Two of the mothers in this study had babies under 2 months of age. However it is interesting to note that each reported that they were coping effectively, and the babies of each were second children.

"Parents are not made at birth, but become parents over time", suggests Neven (1996, p. 53). However, parents may gain ideas about parenting from various sources including, (a) exposure to their own parenting, (b) informal tips and ideas gained from relatives, friends and neighbours, (c) formal education, such as parenting books and health professionals (Harkness & Super, 1992). The legacy of one's own childhood was reported by Kolar and Soriano's (2000) as evident in the way parents spoke about their mothers and fathers and their own respective approaches to parenting, relevant to both Anglo *and* Vietnamese parents.

7.2.2   Elements of Continuity and Persistence

Coping was often described by the mothers in terms of something that required persistence and determination, "coping is keeping going in your role each day, I agree that's what it is …there's surviving and there's really feeling on top of things, but you have to keep going (Wendy). If a mother was to succeed in the cycle of coping, she needed effort and a degree of persistence to see out results from strategies under trial, as described by Wendy, "but a lot of it's trial and error, and seeing what they do as well".

Persistence in coping may also be related to hardiness, or one's inner strength and ability to face challenges. If one is persistent, positive and hopeful in outlook, then one may be more able to cope in the future when a similar situation arises again. This study did not encompass the mothers' dealings with major life event stressors or resilience. It was limited to coping strategies used to deal with day-to-day events, however, the characteristics of coping with each do seem similar. Empowerment and control result from successful coping experiences. When a mother senses this control, she will feel she can make an impact on the environment by assuming control, making decisions and influencing others (Bruess & Richardson, 1989, p. 68).

Resiliency is the ability to 'bounce back' from a difficult situation. A resilient person is able to:

- withstand adversity
- learn from their experiences, and
- cope confidently with life's challenges.

Resilient mothers might be more likely to demonstrate:

- a positive attitude
- optimism
- an ability to regulate emotions
- view failure as a form of helpful feedback (ReachOut, 2017).

When we're resilient we harness inner strengths, utilise our problem-solving skills and coping abilities, however we can also reach out for help and support when it's needed.

7.2.3 Degrees of Coping Are Due to Context

Feeling as though she was coping at a high or low level was often due to the situation the mother found herself in, or 'context', as explained by Wendy:

> I think a lot of it has to do with context, so where you might be just surviving, is when there's things like sick children, less support from other members of the family, or difficult external demands…where there's less of those demands baby's content, things are going all right externally, it's easier to be in a routine or on a roll.

Coping with situations where she knew the reason for the cause of a particular problem made it easier to cope, compared with situations with a more open ended or mysterious cause:

> We tried lots of different things. It was easy because there was a reason for it. They were sick, it seemed easy to just get up, pat them back to sleep, do what we had to do just to get them back to sleep, give them their dummies or whatever. Then it became, it wasn't sickness, illness-related any more, it was, um, habitual waking, so it kept going for another 2 weeks after they were sick. So in knowing what to do then was hard, so we spent a lot of time on the phone to Karitane and Tresillian, umm…it's hard to come up with answers and know what to do…I was at Tresillian for a week, so they gave me ideas there. That was really good. (Wendy)

A very sick child was nominated as a situation less likely to be coped with at a high level:

> I think if I had a really sick child I think I'd find that really quite difficult, but touch wood, Mitchell's in really good health. I mean he doesn't have any chronic conditions, and he doesn't seem to get sick very often with colds or anything like that…I think I'd find that quite worrying and stressful and draining. (Vanessa)

Young, Dixon-Woods, Findlay, and Heney (2002) suggest that mothers, although not ill themselves, experience many of the consequences of chronic illness when caring for sick family members. They described how biographical disruption begins for mothers when they first notice something wrong with their child, and intensifies with diagnosis, altering their sense of self and their social identity. The diagnosis brings with it a set of new responsibilities and role expectations, including an obligation of 'proximity': being physically close to their child at all times to provide 'comfort' and 'keep watch'.

7.2.4   Strategies Are Non-Static; They Are Adaptable and Ever-Changing

Approximately half the mothers interviewed informed me that coping strategies needed to be changed if they were deemed to be not working effectively. A couple of mothers talked about reviewing their array of strategies, such as Sarah:

> Your strategy's always being changed or reviewed. If you realise things aren't working well all of the time, you might analyse things and say, 'I'm gonna stop doing what I'm doing'…For peace of mind, you're going to try something else. I think they [strategies] change all the time.

Coping strategies were evolutionary by nature, "it's [the coping cycle] an ever-changing, ever-learning experience. Every day brings up a new set of circumstances" (Cynthia). A mother needs to be on 'stand-by' mode because her preferred strategy may require refinement or adjustment, "I think on the whole you sort of do things that work for you, and um, I guess some things do take trial and error" (Vanessa). Or for instance, Phillipa believed that change was inevitable and a feature that needed to be highlighted in the coping cycle:

> Yeah, I agree with that [coping cycle], but I don't think that lasts long because when they're young they change so quickly that as soon as you think you've got them organised, they change. So it [strategy] doesn't last long, and you kind of get caught out if you hang on to it too long, because it worked a month ago, but it doesn't work now.

The age group or category of child (such as, babies, toddlers, pre-school, school or adolescent aged child) affected the type of coping strategy employed. This may be the main reason that coping strategies need to be adaptable, "with different age groups, there's a different set of demands, like getting Natasha off to kindy" (Cynthia). This feature was explained well by Wendy:

> There's always going to be new situations arising and you're going to go through it [the coping cycle] again 'cause you've got changing ages representing different problems…a new range of things, and the strategies you've used aren't relevant any more because the things you used were for a different context, they were for younger children.

7.2.5 High Level of Influence from Children in Upturning or Maintaining Balance

The interviews with the mothers contained rich descriptions of the importance and centrality of children in their lives. This may be why they often mentioned children as being highly influential to outcomes of coping strategies, "but then it's often in the kid's control too, if they're happy, you're happy" (Sarah).

While employing a strategy, all mothers were aware of taking into account the feelings of the child. Any coping strategy had to take the child's welfare into account. If the child was happy, then the mother was happy:

> And then that all boils down to that cycle you've got. If they're happy, you're happy doing what you're doing, they're happy and everything's going to go smoothly. You'll try it [the coping strategy] for a little while, and you'll know the results because, for example, you'll feel like things are getting done, and the children are more happy. (Trish)

In most situations, tasks could be made more difficult through the temperament or tiredness level of the child, as explained by these two mothers:

> I think the child's temperament has a lot to do with it. And I think the 'first child syndrome', you know, you give your all, and it was pretty intense with Natasha, I was always quite protective, but I think she is pretty high-maintenance as well. That was really nightmarish, really, when Susanne came. I couldn't believe it, I don't think anyone prepared me for her behaviour. I think just the tantrums when I was breastfeeding and I think almost all of the time. (Cynthia)
>
> …If I'd had Robert as my second child, and he was the difficult baby, I don't think I would have coped at all I think. If you've got a difficult baby like Robert was, it just changes your whole outlook on parenthood. (Sarah)

One minute the mothers could feel they were coping at a high level, and then a new situation would make the mothers feel less adequate:

> It doesn't take a lot to be out of control. Robert will get upset about something and Michelle may have a cold; it will just take something to make the wheels go out of control. (Sarah)

7.2.6 Other Conditions Interfering with Effective Coping

Cynthia recommended against consumption of alcohol at night as a means of coping, as she found she was less effective in her role:

> The glass of wine! I can see how that can be really appealing. Well, I started having a beer with Stephen, and sometimes I'd have a beer when he wasn't here, but then I'd see how it affected me, because often I'd have to do things, like into the night, like paying the bills, or getting things organised, and I couldn't function after one beer. I'd find fatigue hits you then. But I think it depends on your situation.

A few of the mothers mentioned moods and perceptions as affecting their coping; as described by Vanessa, "…but obviously Mitchell has moods, I have moods, Mark has moods, and if Mitchell and I are in a bad mood on the same day, then look out by 5 o'clock!" (Vanessa). It was viewed that extreme negative mood, like postnatal depression, would negatively affect a person's perception of coping outcomes:

> I haven't really though about worrying about coping. I do know one person… I think she's had PND. She tends to always think, 'I'm doing the wrong thing, anyway', and she's the only one I know who thinks, 'I'm a terrible mother'. (Trish)

Trish also felt that she would not cope as effectively if she experienced financial worries:

> I guess if you had financial worries, or you had to worry about other people, or you had to go to work, then I think it would be very hard. But I haven't had anything, I think that's been that drastic. I think being an older parent, I've been lucky, but we planned to work for 'x' amount of years and then, I guess if you're younger you may not be able to plan, and you may find yourself with more financial commitments.

'Additional' activities may push an already stretched mother to overload point, "Any extra activity I find really hard to cope with" (Sarah). It was interesting to note, however, that although Sarah was impressed by mothers who coped *super*-effectively in their roles. However, she wasn't 100% certain "she wanted to go there". It seems she had made a conscious choice not to become a *supermum* or go overboard in fulfilling her role:

> I'm really impressed with mothers who can be out the door and have their washing on the line and their house cleaned before they go. God, they must be up at the crack of dawn. Like I'm not that enthusiastic, and I don't want to go there.

7.3 Learning to Cope and Be Resilient

As a mother faces a particular challenge, such as a tantrumming child or having to complete all of the housework in half a day, she needs to utilise some sort of coping strategy. At early stages of mothering, this may involve trial and error, depending on the amount of prior instruction and advice the mother has received, for example discipline, breastfeeding, or nappy changing methods. After a mother selects her strategy, she implements it, then evaluates whether she feels it has been effective or not. If the strategy doesn't work, the mother will keep trying other methods out, or seek help. Occasionally she may abandon efforts, and do something else more enjoyable, to maintain quality of life (and at times, her sanity!). If the strategy does work, she will feel more assured and in control. She will feel like she is coping. She gains confidence in the knowledge that if a similar situation arises, she can try out her 'proven' strategy. Mothers who face similar situations on repeated occasions become more experienced and confident at taking on a particular type of task or challenge.

The features of the Coping Cycle presented in Fig. 6.1 in Chap. 6 highly resemble the Stages of Learning theory presented in the motor learning literature (Schmidt & Lee, 1999). An important characteristic of learning motor skills is that all people seem to go through three distinct stages when they acquire new skills, as descibed by Magill (2001, pp. 184, 196).

The Fitts and Posner (1979) model consists of the cognitive, associative and autonomous stages. When the learner, or mother, is new to a task, her cognitive thinking will mainly concentrate on determining appropriate strategies, and dropping ineffective ones. According to Schmidt and Wrisberg (2000, p. 13), in the early stages of learning, the individual is simply trying to 'get the hang of' or gain the basic idea of the concept or movement involved to understand its basic pattern of coordination. In order to do this, individuals must do a considerable amount of problem solving, involving the exercise of cognitive and verbal processes. Unfortunately, one's performance or execution of a skill during the early stages of learning is characterised by considerable inaccuracy, slowness, inconsistency and hesitance through lack of confidence (Schmidt & Wrisberg, 2000, p. 13).

Therefore, in her first attempts in the Coping Cycle, or at the Cognitive Stage of Learning, via process of trial and error, the mother will be focusing on assessing the nature of the problem, or what she has to cope with, and ways of solving it (Rose, 1997; Schmidt & Wrisberg, 2000). "Good strategies are retained, and appropriate ones discarded" (Schmidt & Lee, 1999, p. 360). The mother will try out her selected strategy.

As a mother enters the second or Associative Stage of Learning, she will have moved through the Cycle of Coping several times. She will refine her strategy's execution, and modify it where necessary. She is now capable of detecting errors in its execution and more adaptable to changing environmental conditions (Rose, 1997, p. 151). During this period of refinement, refining stage, the person focuses on performing the skill successfully and being more consistent from one attempt to the next (Magill, 2001, p. 184).

According to Magill (2001, p. 184), after much practice and experience, which can take many years, some people move into the final or Autonomous Stage of Learning. The Autonomous Stage of Learning is characterised by higher performance, greater confidence, consistency, and fewer errors. In response to a challenge or situation, a mother can implement her preferred strategy with ease, skill and accomplishment. A mother will also be capable at this point of multi-tasking, or of doing more than one thing while implementing her selected strategy, such as conducting a conversation at the same time (Rose, 1997, p. 151). The mother is able to implement the strategy or skill *automatically*, that is, perform it with ease, giving the impression that she does not have to pay a great deal of attention or effort to what she is doing (Schmidt & Lee, 1999, p. 361; Schmidt & Wrisberg, 2000, p. 187). A reason why a mother who is very experienced at implementing a particular coping strategy and confident with its efficacy, will be due to her perceived consistency of performance during the Autonomous Stage.

Table 7.1 depicts the motor performance characteristics associated with each stage. Having an effective array of strategies available to implement as a challenging situation arises leads to a degree of hardiness, or a feeling of being able to take on further challenges effectively and confidently. The coping strategies described by the mothers mainly refer to strategies in the physical sense, such as "getting things

Table 7.1 Motor performance characteristics associated with each stage of learning

Cognitive stage	Associative stage	Autonomous stage
[Early Learning] Time continuum →	[Mid-Stage Learning] → →	[Later Learning] → →
Associated motor performance characteristics		
Stiff looking	More relaxed	Automatic
Inaccurate	More accurate	Accurate
Inconsistent	More consistent	Consistent
Slow, halting	More fluid	Fluid
Timid	More confident	Confident
Indecisive	More decisive	Decisive
Rigid	More adaptable	Adaptable
Inefficient	More efficient	Efficient
Many errors	Fewer errors	Able to recognise and correct own errors

done", through completed housework, meal preparation and childcare activities. As the children grow older and require less intensive physical care and restraint from a safety point of view through their own increased independence, the cycle of coping may gain more emphasis on the mother's development of psychological and emotional strategies. Therefore, it is postulated that the simplified nature of the model may have limitations when applied to older children 5–12 years, and teenagers. After all, government information states that parent distress increases 40% when children reach teenage years (NSW Parenting Website, 2002).

7.4 Conclusion

It appears that '100% coping, 24/7' with the motherhood role is not a universal experience. A mother may cope in moderate amounts, or only at the bare minimum the bare minimum, but it doesn't mean she is a failure or her child is at risk. Mothering is difficult and it appears that more could be done to support mothers and give them a break from their on-call roles.

However, there is an underlying social expectation of the importance of successful parenting. This may explain the reluctance by some mothers to admit to not coping, as they fear being labelled as an 'unfit mother' by others. Social critique is a very damaging phenomenon.

When mothers do find their strategies effective and are coping at a high level, they feel great satisfaction from the sense of control that arises. As far as assessing whether a coping strategy worked or not, "at the end of the day" this perception was up to the mother. As Trish reiterated:

> …at the end of the day, what is right, what is wrong…I think most mothers would, [think they've done the right thing] well I think, the rewards that you get still outweigh the outcomes of coping.

Factors which impact on a mother's movement through the Cycle of Coping (Fig. 6.1) to higher levels of coping may include:

- Changing circumstances, hence the need to constantly revise or devise new strategies,
- Effect of a child's behaviour or temperament on a particular day, such as the sick or tantrumming child,
- Knowing the cause of a situation, therefore knowing how to effectively pinpoint a possible solution, compared with a problem with a "mystery" cause,
- Feeling determined to continue trying or persist with coping efforts.

Coping describes any positive forms of behaviour designed to manage the stresses and overwhelming feelings that come with tough situations. Learning and developing positive coping skills helps build resilience and well-being for mothers, helping them bounce back when faced with challenges. Resilience can help protect us from various mental health conditions such as depression and anxiety (Mayo Clinic, 2017). Having the confidence and skills to face, overcome or even be strengthened by the challenges of motherhood is a powerful thing for mothers to learn (Parenting SA, 2010).

Chapter 8 presents the conclusions and recommendations of the book.

References

Bruess, C., & Richardson, G. (1989). *Decisions for health* (3rd ed.). Dubuque, Iowa: WM. C. Brown.

Fitts, P., & Posner, M. L. (1979). *Human Performance*. Connecticut, US: Greenwood.

Harkness, S., & Super, C. (1992). Learning to be an American parent: How cultural models gain directive force. In R. G. D'Andrade & C. Strauss (Eds.), *Human motives and cultural modes* (pp. 163–178). Cambridge: University of Cambridge Press.

Kaitz, M., Chikri, M., Bear-Scharf, L. Nir, T., & Eidelman, A. I. (2000). Effectiveness of primiparae and multiparae at soothing their newborn infants. *Journal of Genetic Psychology, 161,* 203–215.

Kolar, V., & Soriano, G. (2000). *Parenting in Australian Families. A comparative study of Anglo, Torres Strait Islander and Vietnamese families. Research Report No. 5. Australian Institute of Family Studies.* Melbourne: Australian Institute of Family Studies.

Magill, R. A. (2001). *Motor learning. Concepts and applications.* NY: McGraw-Hill.

Mayo Clinic. (2017). *Resilience training.* Retrieved from http://www.mayoclinic.org/tests-procedures/resilience-training/in-depth/resilience/art-20046311.

Mercer, R. (1995). *Becoming a mother. Research on maternal identity from Rubin to the present.* New York: Springer.

Neven, R. S. (1996). *Emotional Milestones.* Melbourne: Australian council for educational research Ltd.

NSW Parenting Website. (2002). *NSW parenting campaign.* Sydney: NSW Department of Community Services. Retrieved from http://www.community.nsw.gov.au/document/parent/campaign.pdf.

Parenting South Australia. (2010). *Coping skills. Resilience. Parent easy guide 18.* Adelaide: Children, Youth and Women's Health Service, Department of Health, Government of South Australia.

ReachOut.com. (2017). *Coping skills, resilience.* Retrieved from https://parents.au.reachout.com/skills-to-build/wellbeing/coping-skills-resilience-and-teenagers.

Rose, D. J. (1997). *A multilevel approach to the study of motor control and learning.* Boston, MA: Allyn & Bacon.

Rowe, L., Temple, S., & Hawthorne, G. (1996). Mothers' emotional needs and difficulties after childbirth. Clinical Psychologist, 25, s53–s 58.

Schmidt, R. A., & Lee, T. D. (1999). *Motor control and learning. A behavioral emphasis*. Champaign, IL: Human Kinetics.

Schmidt, R. A., & Wrisberg, C. A. (2000). *Motor learning and performance* (2nd ed.). Champaign, IL: Human Kinetics.

Sethi, S. (1995). The dialectic in becoming a mother: Experiencing a postpartum phenomenon. *Scandinavian Journal of Caring Science, 9,* 235–244.

Tarkka, M.-T., Paunonen, M., & Laippala, P. (1996). Social support provided by nurses to recent mothers on a maternity ward. *Journal of Advanced Nursing, 23,* 1202–1206.

World Health Organisation. (2014). *Mental health. A state of well-being*. Retrieved from http://www.who.int/features/factfiles/mental_health/en/.

Young, B., Dixon-Woods, M., Findlay, M., & Heney, D. (2002). Parenting in a crisis: conceptualising mothers of children with cancer. *Social Science and Medicine, 55,* 1835–1847.

Younger, J. B. (1991). A model of parenting stress. *Research in Nursing & Health, 14,* 197–204.

Chapter 8
Conclusion

Abstract Coping with the challenges of managing motherhood is a positive construct which equates with a mother feeling a greater sense of being in control. Access to strategies usually includes those which incur the least amount of reciprocal obligation. Implementing a successful strategy allows a mother to gain greater confidence and efficacy in that strategy working again for her in future. However, with evolutionary shifts in the changing nature of families, an updated view of examining the contributory role of all family members to its well-being is worth examination so mothers can access further support in their role. Mothers should not have to be responsible for all the childcare and this book has shown that strategies such as help-seeking can do much to ease the strain.

8.1 Managing Motherhood: Summary of the Major Findings

This book has provided a unique insight to mothers' coping experiences. A comprehensive understanding has been achieved of:

1. The meaning of the perceived coping experience
2. Examples of typical situations and demands mothers perceive they have to cope with
3. The main strategies mothers use to cope with these challenges.

In writing this book, I set out to explore the strategies mothers of children 0–5 years utilised in order to cope with their everyday lifestyle, using a grounded theory approach.

The qualitative data revealed the mothers' own subjective points of view and provided their own explanations for any coping experiences. Chapter 4 revealed descriptions of typical coping experiences. The mothers viewed this as a positive

J. L. Currie, *Managing Motherhood*, SpringerBriefs in Well-Being and Quality of Life Research, https://doi.org/10.1007/978-981-13-0338-8_8

sense of feeling in control. They also acknowledged the existence of different degrees of coping, that is, higher and lower levels of coping.

The general nature of the stressors or trigger events leading to coping experiences included pressure to appear as coping; an ideal mother image, lifestyle changes since the baby was born, and the difficulty of the mothering role. Chapter 5 presented the three main categories to emerge from the analysis of the qualitative data clearly indicating key coping methods. Obtaining outside help, having a plan or routine and time-out or escape from normal duties were described by the mothers as methods helping them cope with these situations and to feel in greater control.

Chapters 6 and 7 discussed the implications of the main findings and conditions for effective coping. For the mothers, the process of coping can be difficult to achieve due to it requiring continuous and persistent effort. However, I documented in Chap. 7 how the outcome of coping efforts may be affected by context, or the situational factors involved. Coping strategies were described as being non-static: they are adaptable and ever-changing. Children were noted as being pivotal in upturning or maintaining balance. However, the longer you have been a mother was nominated as making it easier to cope.

8.2   The Theoretical Significance of the Research

The evidence presented in this book supports the notion of coping being health promoting in that it is equivalent to feeling in greater control (McMurray, 2003; WHO, 1986). The research has filled a major gap in the literature being the first to apply grounded theory to discover characteristics about the phenomena of how mothers of young children cope.

Figure 8.1 illustrates the main coping strategies reported by the informants. The most accessible strategies, located closer to the mother in the centre of the circle, include those methods able to be completed by the mother herself. Autonomous strategies, or ones involving the least amount of resources, such as cost free, are also those incorporating the least amount of reciprocal obligation.

To access the qualitative data for this book, the mothers themselves explained to me how they managed motherhood. A cyclic theory on coping was generated from the data, as described in Chap. 6. Implementing a successful strategy allowed a mother to gain greater confidence and efficacy that her strategy would work well again in the future, leading to increased coping and feelings of being in control on a day to day basis.

The theoretical significance includes that the finding that the trial and discovery of successful coping strategies was related to reported subjective wellness by the mothers. Having a strategy on hand meant that the mother tended to feel in greater control of her day to day existence or lifestyle. Coping results

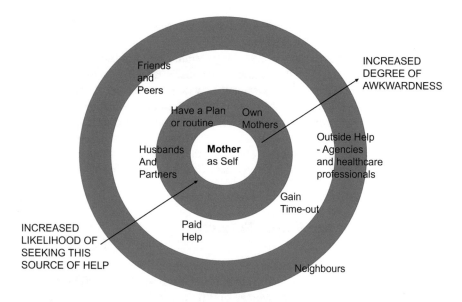

Fig. 8.1 Coping strategies used for managing motherhood

in increased feelings of enjoyment and well-being in the mothering role. Reflecting the philosophy of health promotion, higher levels of health and well-being are characterised by increased control by individuals over their own health, lifestyle and environment (Tones, 1993, p. 7).

One could be forgiven in thinking that parenting is, or *should* be an easy task, given the current plethora of government policies, websites, posters, newspaper items, brochures and so on, educating parents about raising happy child/ren. While this community education material is helpful and points to examples of strategies to cope with difficult children, bedwetting, or death in the family, it is very child-focused, and doesn't describe how normal it is for parents to feel tired, grumpy or not in total control at times, and their need to take a break, for instance. It is also 'OK' for a mother not to be perfect, and my book has shown that different levels of coping are acceptable.

Managing Motherhood is informed by research findings on coping from the parent's point of view. Coping is positive. Coping is a personal achievement contributing to individual mental health. From a new wellness perspective, this book has proposed a new way of defining coping for mothers that is woman-centred and focuses on subjective well-being.

Current parenting education literature and policies aimed at individuals could be described as partially victim-blaming. Health promotion challenges the medicalisation of health, which relies on an ideology blaming each person for their own state of health.

Rather, the social circumstances and people's environment need to be taken into account (Eckersley, Dixon, & Douglas, 2002).

This book challenges the bulk of the coping literature reporting on effective coping which is based on the externally assessed, quantitative inventories. Mothers do not require a clinical expert to medically evaluate how well they feel the mother is coping. This is, in fact, the evaluator's subjective imposition of an external measure on the mother. All that should matter is whether the mother herself feels as if she is coping and can report those perceptions and experiences in her own words. Grounded theory methodology stresses the importance of gaining the mother's perspective, rather than imposing on mothers the researcher's pre-conceived notions of what it means to cope.

8.3 Limitations and Future Research

This book is limited to examining the coping strategies used by a group of five middle-class mothers. However, to broaden recommendations it would be useful for similar research to be conducted with on women of different socio-economic backgrounds including, Culturally and Linguistically Diverse, Indigenous, mothers of disabled children, mothers with a disability, single mothers, grandmothers, younger mothers or employed mothers. The conditions and contexts for effective coping expressed by this group of mothers also needs to be confirmed by others from wider ranging socio-economic backgrounds.

Future research may examine the contribution of fathers and partners to the responsibility for childcare, and their own coping experiences with parenthood. With traditional boundaries, families and parenting evolving and shifting through great changes, it would be useful to understand the contributory role of all family members to the coping process and caring needed to nurture families. Sharing the caring can improve mothers' access to leisure time, a recommended coping mechanism.

8.4 Policy Implications

People are the main resource for achieving health. Mothers will be in a better position to achieve their health potential if they can take control of their environment. However, mothers need support to ensure that healthy choices are easier choices. Equity requires access. The informants contributing to this book were older mothers of young children. Two were university educated, and all had been previously engaged in full-time employment, possibly to return at a later date.

Access to effective coping by lower socio-economic groups may be improved via:

- Maintenance and expansion of the Early Childhood Health Centre Scheme
- Increased programs such the free community pram walking groups, providing social support and friendship, especially when many mothers don't have their own mother living nearby.

Such programs must remain community-centred, free of charge and focused on wellness, not risk group-focused, as this stigmatisation will deter women from attending (Currie & Develin, 2002). Further, changes required in true health promotion strategies must be paralleled by changes in policy (Tones, 1993), for example re-orientation of the content of New Mothers Programs taught in Early Childhood Health Centres, and promotion of increased community connectedness.

The mothers acknowledged the tremendous support and help that could be obtainable from one's own mother. For situations when this is not possible, help-lines such as Dial a Mother, or other social support and community groups involving intergenerational mix, could provide access by young, inexperienced or challenged mums to older, experienced mothers and grandmothers able to offer advice, re-assurance, support, companionship or simply a break. Non-reciprocal outside help including free childcare availability at leisure, workplaces, shopping and local community complexes will go far in offering mothers well-deserved respite from their roles.

8.5 Conclusion

This book has provided enlightenment at the micro-level of the meaning of the coping experience in a group of mothers. At the macro-level, society has not yet developed the attitude that mothers should not have to do all of the caring, nor be on call 24 h a day. However, increased awareness by Australian mothers that strategies such as taking time-out will ultimately improve coping, will do much to improve mothers' sense of well-being and control.

References

Currie, J. L., & Develin, E. D. (2002). Stroll your way to well-being: A survey of the perceived benefits, barriers, community support, and stigma associated with pram walking groups designed for new mothers, Sydney, Australia. *Health Care for Women International, 23,* 882–893.
Eckersley, R., Dixon, J., & Douglas, B. (2002). *The social origins of health and well-being.* Melbourne: Cambridge University Press.
McMurray, A. (2003). *Community health and wellness. A sociological approach.* Sydney: Elsevier.
Tones, K. (1993). The theory of health promotion: Implications for nursing. In J. Wilson-Barnett & J. Macleod-Clark (Eds.), *Research in health promotion and nursing* (pp. 3–14). Houndmills, UK: Macmillan.
World Health Organisation (WHO). (1986). *Ottawa charter for health promotion.* Geneva: WHO.

Index

© The Author(s) 2018
J. Currie, *Managing Motherhood*, SpringerBriefs in Well-Being and Quality
of Life Research, https://doi.org/10.1007/978-981-13-0338-8

Printed in the United States
By Bookmasters